CAN I EAT AT RIVER'S? COOKBOOK

MAKING PLANT-BASED COOKING FUN, EASY, AND NUTRITIOUS FOR THE FAMILY

AMY HAMILTON AND CHAD MITCHELL

PHOTOGRAPHY BY NICOLE MARIE PHOTOGRAPHY, AMY HAMILTON, & EARL JONES

Can I Eat At River's? Cookbook
Copyright © 2019 by Amy Hamilton

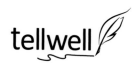

Tellwell Talent
www.tellwell.ca

ISBN
978-0-2288-0813-8 (Hardcover)
978-0-2288-0812-1 (Paperback)

Printed and bound by First Choice Books and Victoria Bindery, in Victoria, BC, Canada

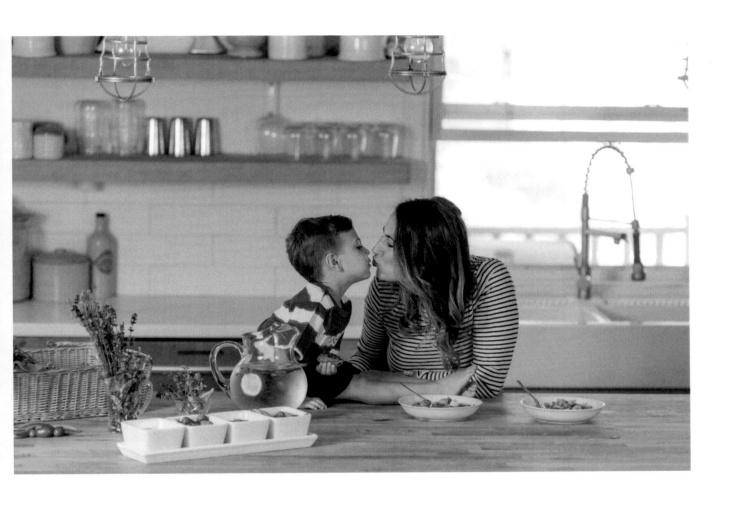

"Let food be thy medicine and medicine be thy food."
-Hippocrates

This book is dedicated to our family
and everyone who helped along the way.

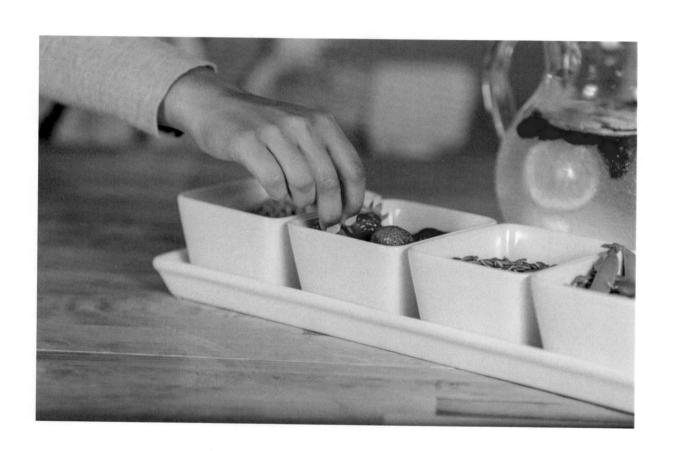

Table of Contents

RISE & SHINE

SAVOURY SIDES

PEACEFUL PLATES

SWEET STREET

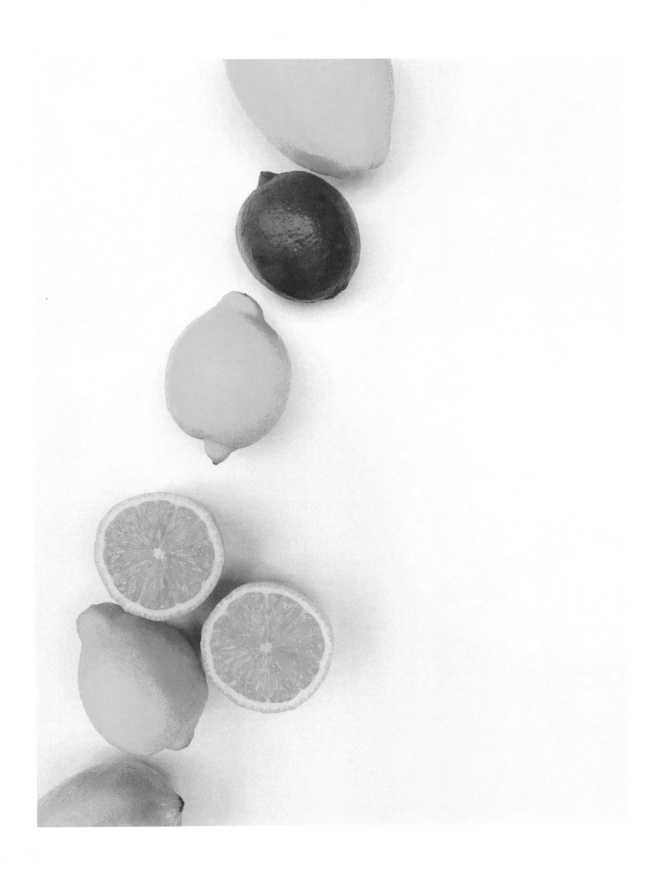

Introduction: Our Family

Our grandmothers are the matriarchs of our families. They showed us how food symbolizes love and unity. Good food is an art form. It evokes our senses and plays with our emotions. Whether we use food to socialize, celebrate our heritage, or simply to fuel our bodies for the day, we can't live without it. However, what we eat makes the difference between getting by and thriving.

While my memories take me back to a small country kitchen in rural Nova Scotia and Chad's to Georgetown, Ontario, we both remember walking into our grandparents' homes and savouring the smell of fresh baked bread while dinner cooked in the oven. We always ate together as a family and shared the food our grandmothers made from scratch. These experiences formed the foundation of our culinary and nutritional educations and helped inspire Chad's desire to become a chef.

As a young child growing up, the world of fine dining was completely foreign to me. I considered a trip to the local Chinese restaurant to be upscale dining. In my early twenties, I began learning more about the healing power of food and how food, especially plants, could be used as preventative medicine. This was a real eye-opener for me that shifted my perspective and approach to cooking. Food needed to be more than just something that tasted good and filled me up. It needed to be nutrient-dense, whole, and as chemically free as possible.

I wasn't just making healthier choices; I felt I was buying health insurance.

When I moved away and met Chad, he introduced me to the world of culinary arts and so began my love affair with fine dining. From the presentation to the social aspect, I was fascinated by all of it. Chad's culinary innovation and passion for creating was something special. He helped further develop my cooking skills and I taught him the things I'd learned about nutrition and how it impacted our health. It was the start of a beautiful partnership.

Along our journey, we became more aware of different agricultural issues and grew passionate about the quality and safety of the food we were preparing. We tried our best to buy organic, local, and non-GMO options as often as possible. We also dabbled with planting our own garden.

When our son, River, was born in 2015, food safety and quality became even more important to us. I was lucky enough to breastfeed him for the first year and make all his baby food. As parents, we have a natural instinct that guides us to make the best choices possible for our children. However, it can be hard to hear the guidance amongst the myriad opinions. I've found the decisions involved in raising River have been the most difficult of my life. When I was in school, globe trotting, or working in the holistic health field, the consequences of my decisions only affected me. Suddenly my choices were so much more important, and it was a lot of pressure! As a health-conscious parent, I started reading and learning more about the benefits associated with a whole foods plant-based diet. The more I learned, the more confident I felt in moving my family towards a significant change.

Making the transition was relativity easy for Chad and I given our backgrounds. Chad was an executive chef working in a high-end private restaurant. I had been a vegetarian in the past and studied holistic health and nutrition. However, when it came to our son, I was fearful. For adults, the research was clear—a well-balanced whole food plant-based diet was healthy and beneficial for possibly reversing or reducing the chances of chronic illness. But there were so many conflicting opinions about raising children on a plant-based diet. Advice came from every direction and I was overwhelmed. I needed to block out the misinformed opinions and trust the science. All research pointed to it not only being safe to raise your child on a plant-based diet but that it was an extremely healthy option.

It was the right decision. During River's routine check-ups at 15 and 18 months we noticed his growth and weight had taken a dip below the normal growth curve for his age group. During this time, we were eating a lot of meat and animal products. We transitioned towards a vegan diet when River was 20 months old. By his two-year check-up, his growth and weight were back on track and his iron levels fell in the healthy, normal range.

River's pediatrician reassured me that whatever I was doing was working and encouraged me to keep it up. To this day he is a healthy, energetic toddler. The only changes that had been made when River was a baby were strictly dietary, primarily plant-based. I say primarily because there were times when he ate fish or something with animal by-products. I found it hard to ensure he was eating strictly vegan when we were travelling or with our families. We were 90 % plant-based and 10 % go with the flow.

I had trouble finding clear guidelines specifically for children's nutritional requirements and meal plans to support a whole foods plant-based diet. This is where inspiration for the cookbook came. I began compiling the nutritional information and Chad helped with recipe development. We wanted to compile everyday meals with clear nutritional labels to inspire parents while sharing favourite recipes and experiences that worked for our family. We also wanted a reference for parents looking to incorporate more healthy meals that the entire family will enjoy.

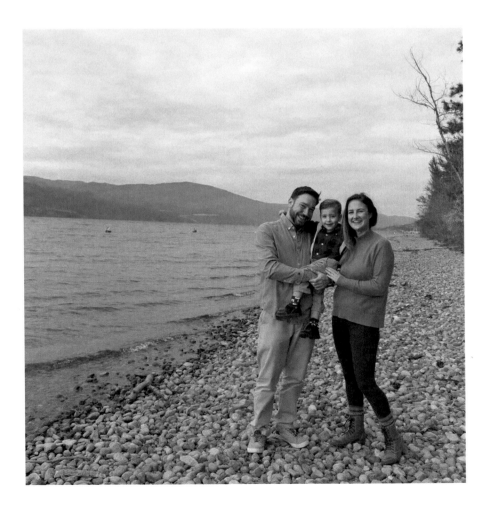

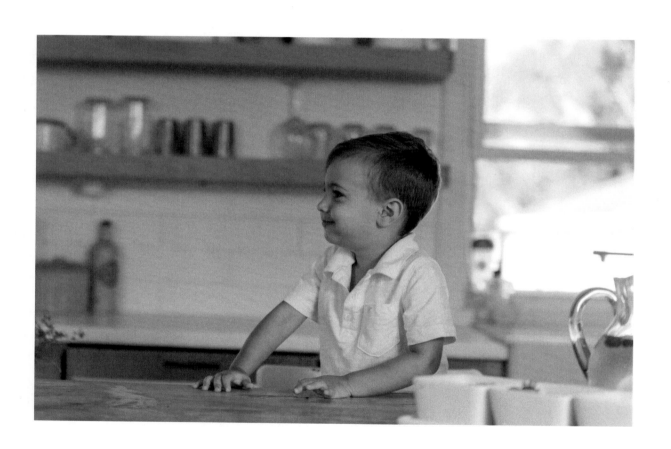

Tips & Tricks

When children and parents are educated about healthy foods, they are empowered to make the best choices. We wanted to lay an early foundation for healthy eating habits with River, in hopes they will stay with him through adulthood.

Children can be fussy with what they will eat; relax, it's normal. What your child may like one day, he or she may not the next. Try to stay cool and never force a child to eat. Mealtime should be fun. You could let them play with their food or eat off your plate. This is a trick that worked well in our household. Remember: monkey see, monkey do.

If River will not eat something I have made, I dish up a plate and start eating. His curiosity will draw him towards me and most of the time he will want to try what I am eating. Sometimes he loves it and we will share; other times he spits it out, which is fine too. My goal is for him to try it. Stay persistent and keep trying to introduce new foods. It can take up to ten taste tests before a child will like a new food.[1,2]

The best way to develop your child's palate is early exposure to a wide variety of foods. I have never shied away from lots of flavour and spice. I don't believe in making a separate meal for the kids. What's for dinner is a meal for the entire family. Our diet includes fruits, vegetables, whole grains, legumes, nuts, and seeds. These foods are rich in phytonutrients, micronutrients, and antioxidants to support a healthy lifestyle.

Being vegan refers to a lifestyle and diet free from animal products. For example, no meat, dairy, honey, eggs, wool, leather, furs, non-vegan make-up, perfume, and soap. A vegan diet doesn't automatically mean it's healthy and well balanced; a vegan could eat Oreos and French fries all day.

When River was young we ate a lot of soups, chilies, and curries, anything that was easy to purée for him. If it needed to be seasoned more for the adults, we just set aside a portion for River, and seasoned ours separately. Since we make pretty much everything from scratch it can take a little more time, so we make large batches and freeze the leftovers. This way we are not in the kitchen every day for hours at a time. This was especially important when we were working away from the house full-time.

Now that River is a little older, he wants to help me in the kitchen. I encourage him by having him pull up a chair and get involved as much as possible, from pouring liquids into the bowl and stirring, to taste-testing.

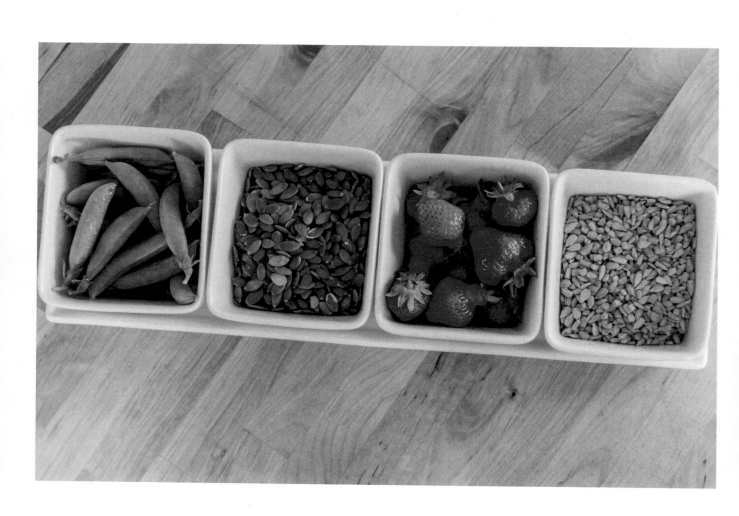

The Basics: What you need to know when eating a plant-based diet

The most important thing to be aware of with a plant-based diet is making sure you are getting enough B12, since it is the only vitamin acquired through animal products. B12 is important for proper metabolism, it forms DNA, and it keep nerves working properly.[3] Some products are fortified with B12 but check the labels to be sure. You might want to consider a B12 supplement or a good multivitamin for your child.

Zinc and Iron are also worth paying attention to. Zinc is important for skin health and it strengthens the immune system.[4] Iron ensures proper hemoglobin production and circulation of oxygen in the blood. If your child is having non-heme sourced iron (meaning it doesn't come from animals), he or she will need to consume double the amount on a plant-based diet since it doesn't absorb as well as the heme iron. It is important to include Vitamin C when eating non-heme iron sources. Vitamin C will increase the absorption of the non-heme iron.[5] Also, cooking in a cast iron skillet will enrich your foods with iron.

Fats are really important for brain development, especially in the first three years.[6] There are lots of healthy plant-sourced fats. Omega 3s are composed of three types: ALA (alpha-linolenic acid), DHA (docosahexaenoic acid), and EPA (eicosapentaenoic acid). ALA is an essential fatty acid, meaning your body doesn't make it; therefore, it needs to be consumed in the diet. Our bodies can turn ALA into DHA and EPA but not very well.[7] For this reason, we supplement with an algae oil that contains DHA and EPA.

Vitamin D improves bone density and mental health, it helps absorb calcium, and it supports the immune system.[8] Vitamin D can be fortified in products. Read the labels to be sure. Your skin will also make Vitamin D when it is exposed to sunlight.

Calcium helps build healthy bones and teeth.[9] There are lots of plant sources of Calcium and it is often fortified in products as well.

Most people don't include Iodine, but I do, since we don't eat seafood. Iodine is a component of two thyroid hormones that help regulate growth, development, and metabolism.[1, 10, 11, 12]

	B12	Vitamin D	Calcium	Iron	Zinc	Iodine	Fats
Food Sources	fortified in food such as soy milk, Red Star & Braggs Nutritional Yeast	fortified in non-dairy milks & sunshine	blackstrap molasses, tahini, dark leafy greens, almonds, tofu, & fortified in non-dairy milks	soybeans, lentils, blackstrap molasses, dark leafy greens, tempeh, tofu, tahini, peas, raisins, & watermelon	grains, legumes, nuts, & pumpkin seeds	seaweed, kelp, dulse, nori, & plants grown in iodine rich soil	flaxseed, canola oil, tofu, soybeans, avocado, coconut, chia, algae oil, hemp seeds, nuts, & seeds including butters

1, 3, 4, 5, 7, 8, 9, 10, 11, 12

Carbohydrates

Carbohydrates have gotten a bad name, which isn't accurate. They are not just pasta and breads but fruits and vegetables as well. Children aged one to eight are required to intake 130 grams of carbs per day, which is where they will get a good part of their dietary fibre. Children who are one to three years of age should be getting at least 19 grams of fibre per day. Children four to eight years of age should be getting 25 grams per day. Health Canada found that fibre intake of children in both age groups fell below the recommended amount. A whole foods plant-based diet provides a high fibre intake.[1,3,14]

Proteins

If you are like me, you have probably been caught in the protein craze at some time in your life. Make sure you and your children are getting enough protein. Children aged one to three require 13 grams/day and children four to eight need 19 grams/day.[1,3] How will you get protein if you don't eat meat? Relax, there are lots of plant sources. The body is a miraculous thing. It can take the various incomplete proteins that you eat throughout the day and make them into complementary proteins, which are equivalent to complete proteins. Breast milk, which has the lowest amount of protein when compared to cow's or goat's milk, is perfectly formulated to meet a growing baby's nutritional requirements.[15]

Fats

Fat is crucial for brain development in children and almost half of their caloric intake should come from fat in the first three years.[6] Much of the fat should be sourced from monounsaturated and polyunsaturated fats. Studies found 47% of Canadian children aged one to three were not getting enough fat whereas only 5.5% of children four to eight were not getting enough fat. Children between the ages of one to eight that were getting the recommended amount of fat were consuming more saturated fat than mono and polyunsaturated. Health Canada recommends that the saturated fat intake remain as low as possible.[13]

	B12		Vitamin D		Calcium		Iron		Zinc		Iodine		Omega 3		Folate (Folic Acid)	
	RDA/AI	UL	RDA/AI	UL	RD/AI	UL	RDA/AI	UL	RDA/AI	UL	RDA/AI	UL	AI	UL	RDA/AI	UL
1-3 years old	0.9 micrograms	ND	600 International Units	2500 International units	700 milligrams	2500 milligrams	7 milligrams	40 milligrams	3 milligrams	7 milligrams	90 micrograms	200 micrograms	0.7 grams	ND	150 micrograms	300 micrograms
4-8 years old	1.2 micrograms	ND	600 International Units	3000 International Units	1000 milligrams	2500 milligrams	10 milligrams	40 milligrams	5 milligrams	12 milligrams	90 micrograms	300 micrograms	0.9 grams	ND	200 micrograms	400 micrograms
Pregnancy 19 years and older	2.6 micrograms	ND	600 International Units	4000 International Units	1000 milligrams	2500 milligrams	27 milligrams	45 milligrams	11 milligrams	40 milligrams	220 micrograms	1100 micrograms	1.4 grams	ND	600 micrograms	1000 micrograms
Lactation 19 years and older	2.8 micrograms	ND	600 International Units	4000 International Units	1000 milligrams	2500 milligrams	9 milligrams	45 milligrams	12 milligrams	40 milligrams	290 micrograms	1100 micrograms	1.3 grams	ND	500 micrograms	1000 micrograms
Food Sources	1 cup non-dairy beverage, fortified = 1 mcg; 2 tsp Red Star T6635+ Yeast flakes (Vegetarian Support Formula) = 1 mcg		1 cup rice, oat and almond beverage, fortified = 85-90 IU; ½ cup orange juice, fortified = 50 IU		½ cup spinach, cooked = 129 mg; 1 tbsp blackstrap molasses = 179 mg; 1 cup soy beverage, fortified with calcium = 321-324 mg; 2 tbsp tahini = 130 mg; ¾ cup tofu, prepared with calcium sulfate = 302-525 mg; ¼ cup almonds, dry roasted, unblanched = 93 mg		¾ cup tempeh, cooked = 3.2 mg; ½ cup spinach, cooked = 2-3.4 mg; 1 tbsp blackstrap molasses = 3.6 mg; ¾ cup of lentils, cooked = 4.1-4.9 mg; ¾ cup tofu, cooked = 2.4-8 mg; 1 tbsp sesame seeds roasted = 1.4 mg; ¾ cup peas (chickpeas/garbanzo, black-eyed, split), cooked = 1.9-3.5 mg		¼ cup of pumpkin or squash seeds = 2.7-4.4 mg; ½ cup wild rice, cooked = 1.2 mg; ¾ cup lentils, cooked = 1.9 mg; ¾ cup dried peas (chickpeas/garbanzo beans, black-eyed, split) cooked = 1.1-1.9 mg; 2 tbsp tahini = 1.4 mg		1 gram seaweed = 16-2 984 mcg; 1 slice bread (rye, whole wheat, white) = 17-32 mcg		1 tbsp flax meal = 2.43 g; 1 tbsp chia seeds = 1.9 g; ¼ cup walnuts = 0.85-2.30 g; ¾ cup tofu, cooked = 0.27-0.48 g; ½ cup edamame/baby soybeans, cooked = 0.29-0.34 g; ½ cup radish seeds, sprouted, raw = 0.42 g		¾ cup lentils, cooked = 265 mcg; ½ cup edamame/baby soybeans, cooked = 106-255 mcg; ½ cup spinach, cooked = 121-139 mcg; 4 spears asparagus, cooked = 128-141 mcg; ¾ cup beans (pink, pinto, navy, black, white, kidney, great northern), cooked = 157-218 mcg	

Please note that Recommended Dietary Allowances (RDA) and Adequate Intakes (AI), are the minimum amounts needed to meet sufficient nutritional requirements. UL, indicates tolerable upper intake levels, meaning you want to stay below the UL to avoid adverse health risks. ND means upper intake levels have not been determined. [3, 4, 5, 7, 8, 9, 10,14, 16,17]

Cooking Tips

How to properly prepare nuts and seeds

Nuts and seeds provide many beneficial nutrients and are a fundamental part of a plant-based diet. I don't think it's common knowledge but it's important to properly prepare nuts and seeds. This makes them easier to digest and their nutrients more readily available. This is especially important for children who have immature digestive systems. Nuts and seeds should be soaked in salt water overnight and dried before eating. Here is the basic process:

- Dissolve ½ tbsp of sea salt in approximately 5 cups of water.
- Add 2 cups of nuts.
- Soak for a minimum of 7 hours or overnight.
- Rinse and strain the nuts.
- Preheat oven to no more than 150°F.
- Line a baking sheet with parchment and place nuts on the baking sheet.
- Dry the nuts for 12 to 24 hours in the oven, sun, or dehydrator.
- Cool and store in an airtight container in the fridge or freezer.

Almost all nuts and seeds can be prepared this way expect for flax or chia seeds or any other seed that becomes slimy when soaked.

How to make a vegetable stock

We love to use homemade vegetable stocks as much as we can. It is a great alternative to store-bought stock, especially if you are watching your sodium intake. To make a vegetable stock, save all vegetables and herb trimmings in the fridge in an airtight container, except for potatoes or any vegetables which are high in starch (starches will affect the clarity of the stock). Once you have about two or three cups worth, fill a large pot with water and add your trimmings, peppercorns, and a couple of bay leaves. Simmer with the lid off for 45 minutes to an hour. Once it is finished, strain off and set stock aside to cool. If you don't use it right away, store in an airtight container in the fridge for three or four days or freeze. Stocks are great for soups, broths, and cooking grains. We also like to make different types of stocks depending on the dish we are creating. We like to use fresh ginger, star anise, mushroom stalks, kelp, and oranges for making Asian broths or dashi. We use fresh herbs and stems that are native to the regions.

Cooking tips for beans

We buy dry beans in bulk. It is more cost-effective than buying canned beans. We still keep canned beans on hand for when we are in a hurry and don't have time to cook the dry beans. When you are eating a plant-based diet beans become a staple. If you soak your beans overnight, for seven to twelve hours, they will cook faster and become easier to digest. One cup of dry beans yields approximately 2 ¼ cups of cooked beans. If you want to avoid the gassiness associated with beans and make them even more digestible, drain and rinse the beans after the first boil when a foam starts to appear on the top. Add new water and continue to cook. Once the beans have finished cooking, strain, and rinse with cool water. Beans can last approximately three to four days in the refrigerator once cooked.

Cooking Times for Legumes and Grains		
1 Cup	Cook Time	Amount of Water
All beans should be soaked overnight in water for 7-12 hours before being cooked.		
Black Beans*	45-60 minutes	6 cups
Chickpeas or Garbanzo*	75-90 minutes	6 cups
Kidney & White Beans*	70-90 minutes	6 cups
Everything below does not need to be soaked. When cooking all types of rice, rinse first. After cooking rice, remove from heat, cover, let stand for 5 minutes and then fluff with a fork.		
Green, French, red and yellow lentils*	15-20 minutes	3 cups
Green and yellow split peas*	40-60 minutes	3 cups
Quinoa*	15-20 minutes	2 cups
Brown Rice (short and long grain)*	30 minutes	2 ¼ cups
White Basmati*	15 minutes	2 cups
Brown Basmati*	25 minutes	2 cups
Sushi Rice*	10-15 minutes	1 cup
Old Fashioned Rolled Oats	10-15 minutes	2 cups
Quick Oats	5 minutes	2 cups
* Gluten-free		
Rolled and Quick Oats can be substituted for gluten-free options.		

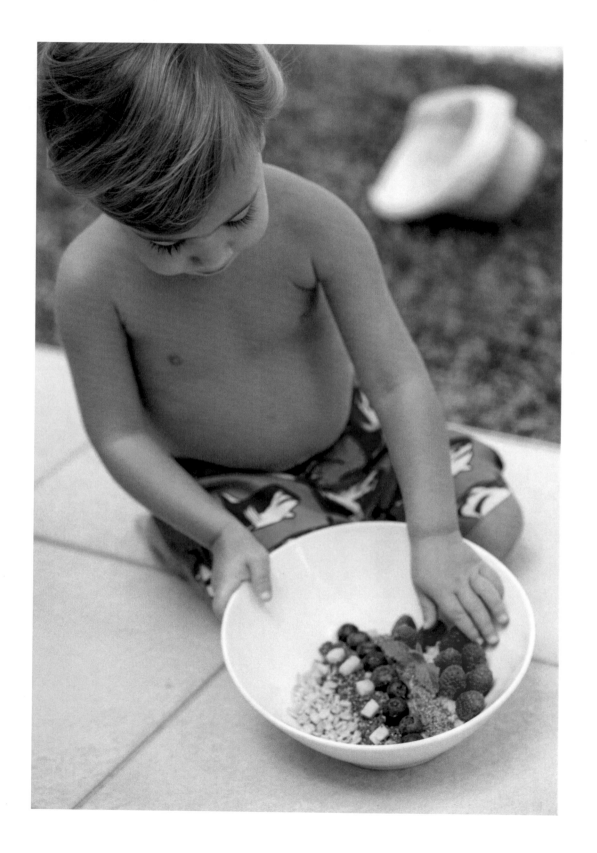

RISE &
SHINE

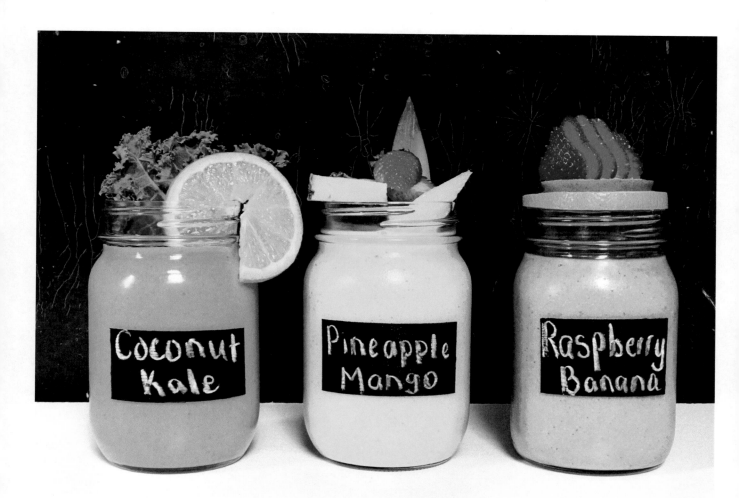

Smoothie Operator

Smoothies are great for many things in our household, whether it's to make up for breakfast when running behind, or a way to sneak greens and added nutrients into River, especially if he is having an off day. With all the nuts, seeds, fruit, and avocado, it almost becomes a meal in a glass. It can also come in handy in the heat of the summer as quick meal replacer in the morning.

Gluten-free   Ready in 5 minutes   Serves 4

Coconut Kale & Banana

1 cup non-dairy milk
1 ½ cups can coconut milk
½ cup ice
2 cups packed kale
1 banana
½ avocado
1 tbsp agave nectar
3 tbsp hemp seeds

Mango-Pineapple

2 cups non-dairy milk
1 cup mango juice
½ cups non-dairy yogurt
1 cup greens (optional)
1 ½ cups frozen mangoes
1 cup fresh pineapple
2 tbsp flax meal
2 tbsp chia seeds

Raspberry-Banana

2 cups non-dairy milk
¾ cup orange juice
1 banana
1 ½ cups raspberries
½ avocado
2 tbsp flax meal
2 tbsp hemp seeds

For all smoothies place all ingredients into a blender, purée, and serve.

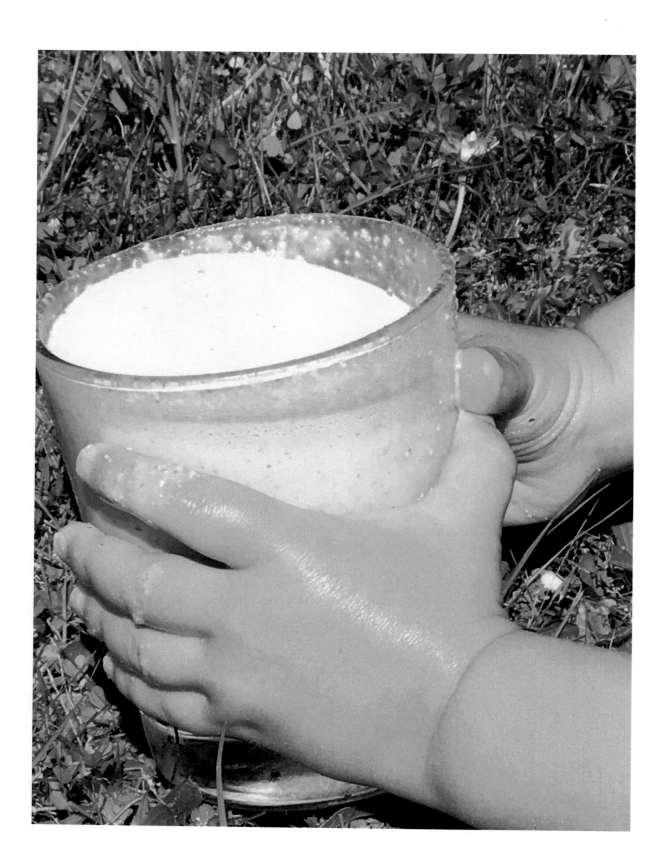

Peanut Butter Smoothie

This smoothie is comparable to a milkshake. It is one of River's favourites. The walnuts and pumpkin seeds provide healthy fats as well as zinc. Try adding a handful of greens, to sneak in an extra nutritional boost.

Gluten-free   Ready in 5 minutes   Serves 4

3 cups non-dairy milk
1 ripe banana
½ cup walnuts
¼ cup pumpkin seeds
2 tbsp flax meal
2 tbsp peanut butter
pinch of nutmeg
½ cup ice

Place all ingredients into the blender and purée. Adding ½ cup of ice helps keep the smoothie nice and chilled on warmer days if needed.

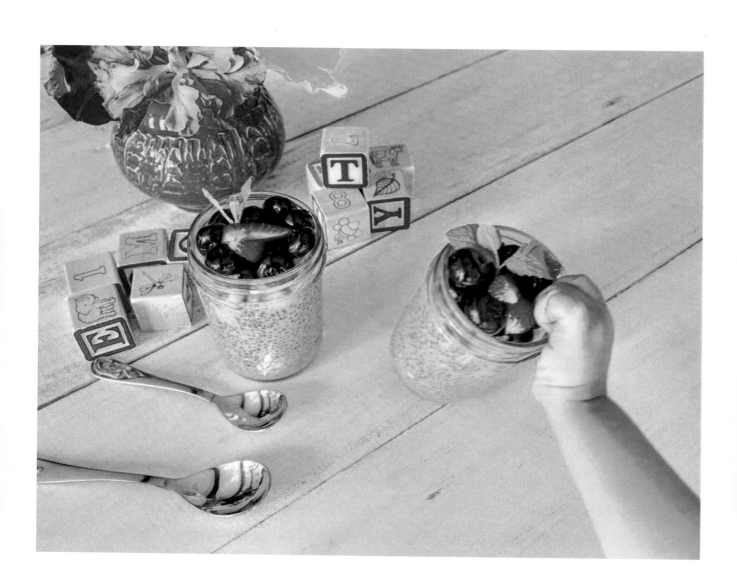

Cha Cha-Chai-Chia Seed Pudding

We love the flavours of a good chai latte and the ease with which this neat little pudding comes together. Waking up the next day and adding some diced mango or fresh berries from the yard turns this simple pudding into a fun, sweet snack for all.

Gluten-free   Ready in 5–6 hours   Serves 2

1 ½ cups vanilla soy milk or non-dairy milk
4 tbsp chia seeds
¼ tsp ginger powder
¼ tsp cardamom, ground
½ tsp cinnamon
pinch of cloves
⅛ tsp nutmeg

In a small saucepan on low heat add milk and spices. Whisk and let infuse for 5 minutes.

Pour the milk and spices into a small bowl. Whisk in chia seeds and let set in the refrigerator overnight or 4–5 hours.

Garnish with fruit and serve.

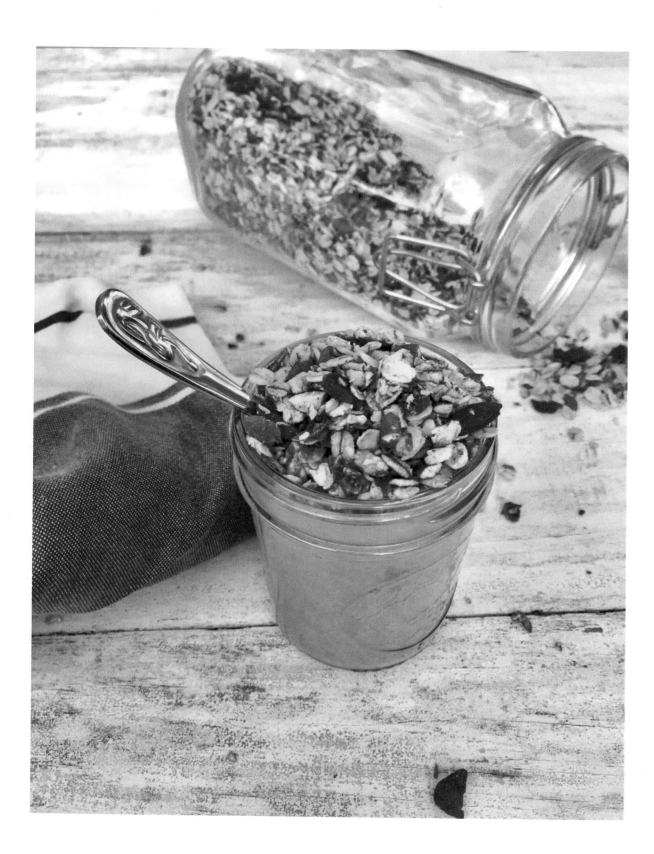

Goji Berry Granola & Yogurt

When it comes to summer mornings and early snacks, what goes better with cool and crisp coconut yogurt than crunchy, delicious granola and dried fruits folded in? The goji berries are great to use not just for keeping things interesting and different, but they are delicious and very high in Vitamin C. The granola stores well and can be kept fresh on hand in a mason jar or Ziploc bag.

Gluten-free   Ready in 25 minutes   Makes 3 ¼ cups Granola

1 ½ cups rolled oats, gluten-free
¾ cup shredded unsweetened coconut
⅓ cup pumpkin seeds
½ cup almonds, chopped
⅓ cup goji berries
3 tbsp coconut oil
¼ cup maple syrup
¾ tsp cinnamon
¼ tsp nutmeg
dash of sea salt

Preheat oven to 350°F. Line a baking tray with parchment paper.

In a large mixing bowl combine rolled oats, shredded coconut, pumpkin seeds, almonds, cinnamon, nutmeg, and sea salt. Mix together.

In a small pot over low heat melt the coconut oil and whisk in the maple syrup. Pour liquid mixture over dry mixture. Stir well.

Pour mixture on the lined baking tray and spread evenly. Bake for 15 minutes then remove from oven and stir. Put back in the oven for an additional 3–5 minutes until golden brown. Remove from oven and allow to cool.

Stir in goji berries after granola has baked and cooled. Serve over yogurt. One serving of granola equals ¼ cup.

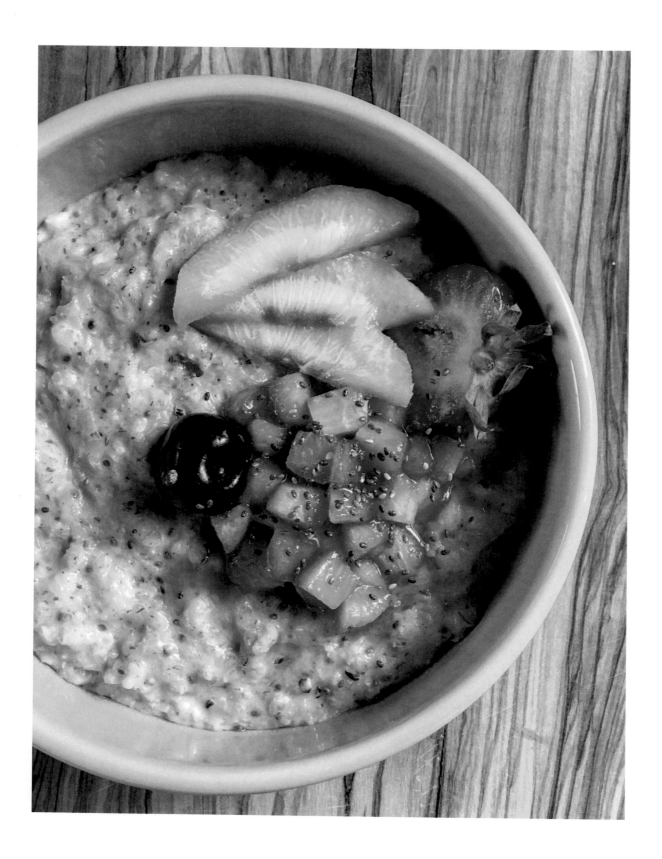

Wild Oatsmeal

Growing up, oatmeal was breakfast 3 or 4 days a week, so it got boring at times. Using different fruits and spices makes it more fun for all of us. Living in British Columbia we try to can and preserve all the beautiful fruit that surrounds us when fall comes, like peaches, pears, plums, cherries, and apples. Then we add it to our oatmeal all winter.

Gluten-free   Ready in 6–10 minutes   Serves 2

Peaches 'n' Cream Oatmeal

½ cup quick oats, gluten-free
1 cup water
1 peach, peeled and diced
dash of cinnamon
1 tsp cane sugar
1 tbsp flax meal
1 tbsp hemp seeds
1 tbsp chia seeds
⅔ cup soy milk or non-dairy milk

Blueberry Oatmeal

½ cup quick oats, gluten-free
1 cup water
½ cup blueberries
dash of cinnamon
1 tbsp flax meal
1 tbsp hemp seeds
1 tbsp chia seeds
⅔ cup soy milk or non-dairy milk

Peaches 'n' Cream

In a medium pot bring water to a boil. Then add oatmeal. See cooking chart on page xix.

In a small frying pan add peaches and cane sugar and reduce, gently crushing peaches to release the juices. Sauté for 4–5 minutes until peaches caramelize.

Add peaches, flax meal, chia seeds, hemp seeds, and cinnamon to oatmeal. Add milk, stir, and serve.

Blueberry

In a medium pot bring water to a boil. Then add oatmeal. See cooking chart on page xix.

Add blueberries, flax meal, chia seeds, hemp seeds, and cinnamon to oatmeal. Add milk, stir, and serve.

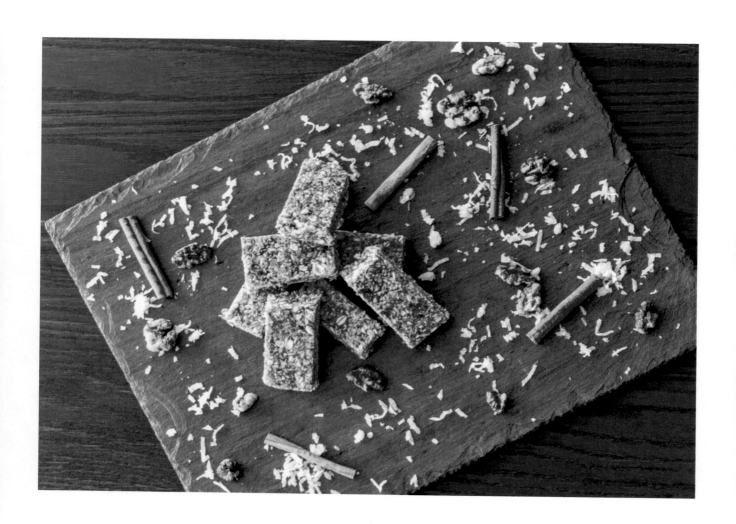

Maple-Nut Granola Bars

When in doubt pack snacks for throughout. Packing snacks and being prepared for extended travels or trips is a life-saver. Whether to prevent meltdowns or just to keep those hunger cravings in check, we always have enough for all three of us. Once these are prepared they are great to set out for gatherings or to individually portion and wrap for packed lunches or travel. Either way, we always find plenty of ways to make them disappear.

Gluten-free   Ready in 2 hours 15 minutes   Makes 16 Bars

¾ cup peanut butter, almond butter, or tahini
¼ cup coconut oil
½ cup maple syrup
1 ¾ cups quick oats, gluten-free
½ cup flax meal
1 cup shredded unsweetened coconut
½ cup almonds
½ cup walnuts
½ tsp cinnamon
½ tsp sea salt
1 ½ tsp vanilla

In a small saucepan over low heat add coconut oil, maple syrup, peanut butter, and vanilla. Stir together until everything is well mixed. Remove from heat.

In a blender or food processor pulse the almonds and walnuts until finely ground. Finely grinding the nuts prevents children from choking on large pieces.

In a medium mixing bowl mix quick oats (if you have rolled oats just give them a quick pulse in the food processor to crumble), flax meal, shredded coconut, cinnamon, sea salt, ground almonds, and walnuts.

Add coconut oil, maple syrup, and peanut butter mixture in the medium bowl with dry ingredients and mix together.

Line a 9" x 9" baking dish with parchment paper. With a wooden spoon, pour granola bar mixture into the baking dish. Take a small piece of parchment paper and press down the mixture until it is flat and even.

Cover and place the bars in the fridge for 2 hours or overnight.

When ready to cut bars, lift the parchment out of the baking dish, cut bars into 16 pieces, and enjoy. Store in airtight container in the fridge. One serving equals one bar.

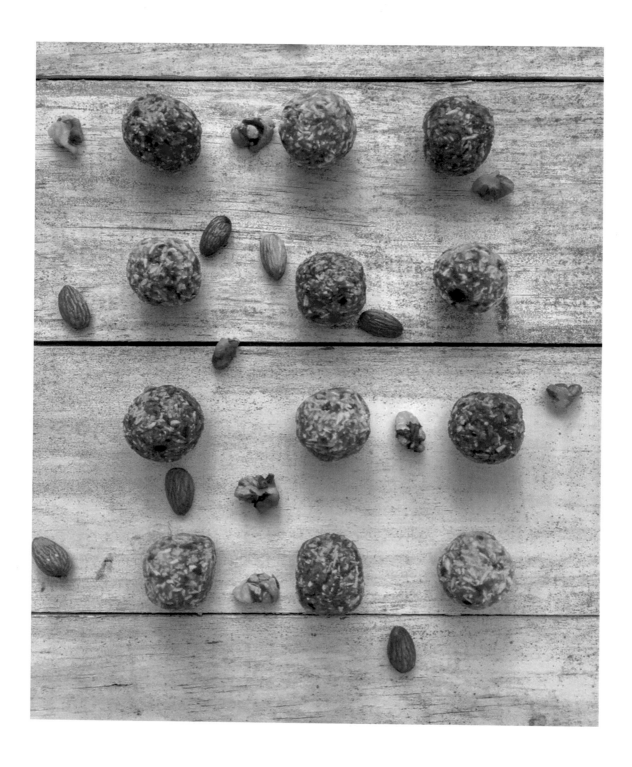

High-Energy Bites

These bite-sized snacks offer a quick burst of energy or a boost to help the body quickly replenish when feeling drained. Hidden in a pocket or packed for a mid-afternoon nosh, these tasty snacks are a nice no baking or cooking crowd pleaser.

Gluten-free   Ready in 30 minutes   Makes 8 Bites

Carrot Cake

½ cup quick oats or rolled oats, gluten-free
⅓ cup shredded unsweetened coconut
½ cup shredded carrot
½ cup walnuts
½ cup dates
½ tsp cinnamon
pinch nutmeg
¼ tsp ginger powder
pinch of sea salt

Lemon Zinger

½ cup quick oats or rolled oats, gluten-free
⅓ cup shredded unsweetened coconut
½ cup sunflower seeds
½ cup dates
zest of one lemon
¼ tsp turmeric
pinch of sea salt

Carrot Cake High-Energy Bites

Soak dates in warm water for 25 minutes to soften. Strain and remove the pits. Soak walnuts in warm water for 25 minutes and strain.

In a medium bowl add oats (if you are using rolled oats pulse in the food processor to crumble), shredded coconut, grated carrot, cinnamon, nutmeg, ginger, and sea salt; mix together.

In a food processor or mini chop, add dates and walnuts and pulse until a sticky mixture forms.

Add the date and walnut mixture to the dry ingredients and mix together with your hands until you have formed a large ball.

Mould into 8 round balls and serve. Store in an airtight container in fridge. One serving equals one High-Energy Bite.

Lemon Zinger High-Energy Bites

Soak dates in warm water for 25 minutes to soften. Strain and remove the pits. Soak sunflower seeds in warm water for 25 minutes and strain.

In a medium bowl add oats (if you are using rolled oats pulse in the food processor to crumble), shredded coconut, lemon zest, turmeric, and sea salt; mix together.

In a food processor or mini chop, add dates and sunflower seeds and pulse until a sticky mixture forms.

Add the date and sunflower mixture to the dry ingredients and mix together with your hands until you have formed a large ball.

Mould into 8 round balls and serve. Store in an airtight container in fridge. One serving equals one High-Energy Bite.

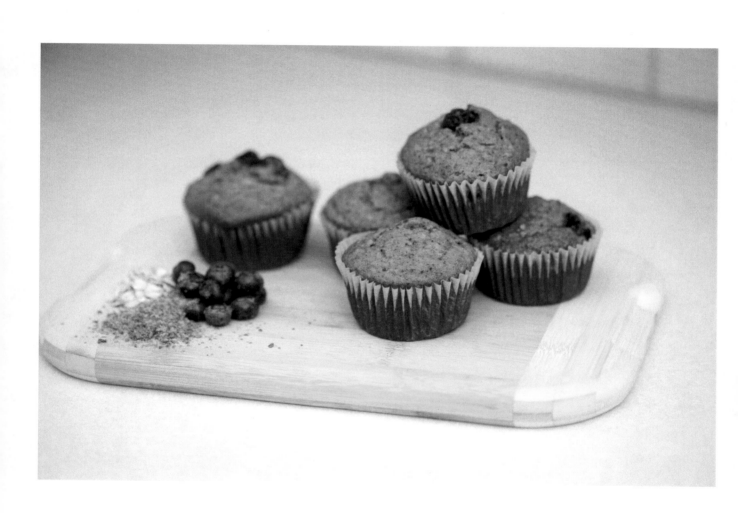

Never "Blue"berry Oatmeal Muffins

Having a tasty, healthy muffin recipe is a must for our household. Whether they're warm out of the oven with a flavoured vegan butter, or even just to grab off the kitchen counter and snack away, these blueberry oatmeal muffins are an awesome way to keep everyone happy.

Ready in 25 minutes   Makes 12 Muffins

1 ½ cups spelt flour
½ cup of rolled oats
1 banana, mashed
1 cup blueberries
¾ cup soy milk or non-dairy milk
2 tbsp flax meal + 6 tbsp water
½ cup of turbinado sugar
¼ cup coconut oil
2 tsp baking soda
pinch of sea salt

Maple Ginger Butter
1 tsp fresh ginger, peeled and grated
1 tbsp maple syrup
½ cup vegan butter
¼ tsp cinnamon

Preheat oven to 350°F. Line muffin pan with muffin cups.

Prepare egg replacer. Mix 2 tbsp of flax meal in 6 tbsp of water and let sit for 5 minutes until it has thickened.

In a large bowl add rolled oats (pulse rolled oats in the food processor until finely ground), sift spelt flour, baking soda (to remove lumps), and sea salt. Mix.

In a medium mixing bowl, purée the banana with a stick blender. Add sugar, oil, egg replacer, and cream together. Then add soy milk.

Pour wet ingredients in with the dry ingredients and mix together. Then fold in blueberries.

Scoop batter into muffin cups and bake for 15 minutes.

While muffins are baking, prepare the Maple Ginger Butter. Place all ingredients into a mixing bowl or electric mixer and beat butter with paddle or ladle, scraping down sides until all ingredients are incorporated and butter is smooth, light, and fluffy. Remove from bowl and reserve for when needed.

Remove from oven and allow to cool. One serving equals one muffin.

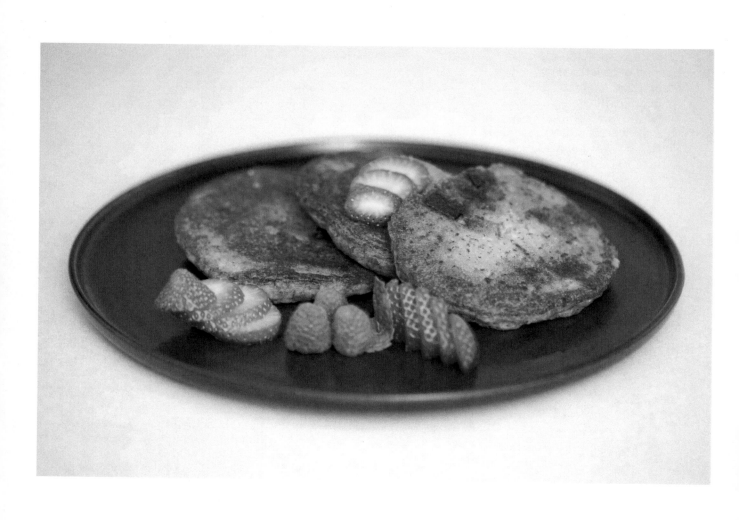

Banana, Coconut, & Chocolate Chip Pancakes

Warm pancakes and maple syrup is a great way to start any day. We love the combination of chocolate and coconut, and the flavour of the banana when it is seared and slightly caramelized in the pan. This was one of the first recipes we developed for ourselves and for the book; it is also one of our most used recipes. Adding lemon and blueberries or other fruits and spices keeps it fun and allows us to introduce more flavour profiles to River.

Ready in 15 minutes   Makes 6 Small Pancakes

1 cup spelt flour
¼ cup shredded unsweetened coconut
¾ cup soy milk or non-dairy milk
1 mashed banana
1 tbsp flax meal + 3 tbsp of water
½ tsp baking soda
1 tbsp coconut oil
2 tbsp coconut oil for cooking
2 tbsp chia or hemp seeds
⅓ cup of vegan chocolate chips (optional)
pinch of salt

Prepare egg replacer. Mix 1 tbsp of flax meal and 3 tbsp of water and let sit for 5 minutes until it has thickened.

In a medium bowl, purée a banana, add milk, 1 tbsp of melted coconut oil, and egg replacer; whisk together. Add spelt flour, baking soda, chia seeds, and shredded coconut into the bowl with the wet ingredients and mix. If batter seems a little dry add a couple more tbsp of milk. The chia seeds will absorb some of the liquid. Once everything is well combined fold in chocolate chips.

Preheat a large frying pan with 1 tbsp of coconut oil over low-medium heat. Pour in pancake batter. Once little bubbles start to appear on the surface of the pancakes flip and fry the other side. Add the extra tbsp of oil as needed for frying. Double the recipe for more than three people.

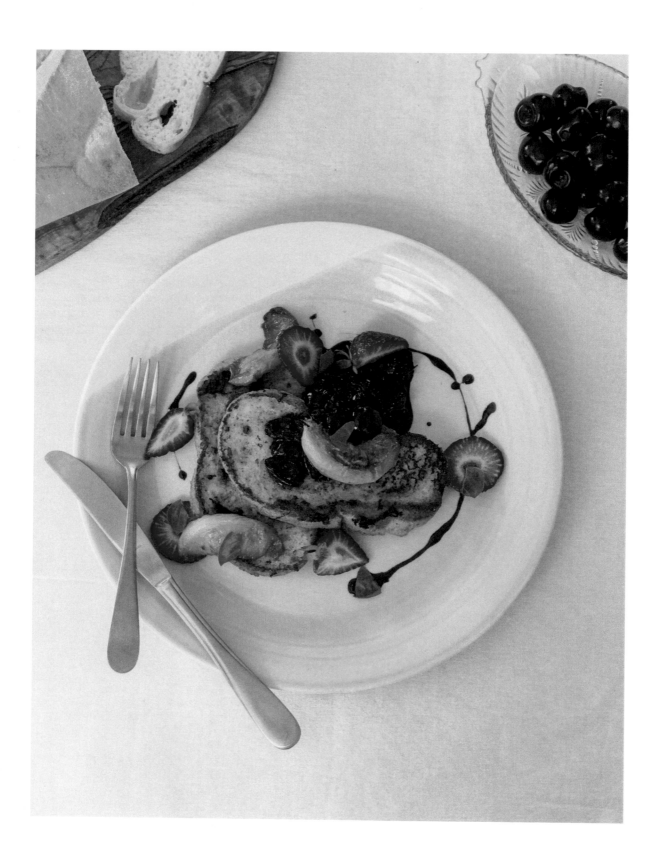

French Toast with Glazed Peaches
&
Cherry Compote

This is a favourite of kids and adults alike! This French toast egg replacer works amazing. It is a great way to use up leftover bread or a great excuse to pick up a fresh loaf from a local bakery. It's just as good on its own with warm syrup as it is with peaches and cherry compote, or any fruit jam or chutney for that matter.

Ready in 25 minutes   Serves 3

1 loaf French bread
2 peaches cut into eighths
2 tbsp maple syrup
1 cup soy milk or non-dairy milk
2 tbsp flax meal
2 bananas
2 tbsp coconut oil

Cherry Compote

1 cup cherries, pitted
½ cup water
3 tsp cane sugar
pinch cinnamon
dash nutmeg
1 tsp cornstarch

Preheat oven to 375°F. Line baking sheet with parchment paper.

Lay peach slices flat on their side. Drizzle with 1 tbsp of maple syrup. Bake for 6–8 minutes. Remove from oven, flip, and glaze the other sides with 1 tbsp of maple syrup. Bake for another 8–10 minutes.

Mix 2 tbsp of flax meal in the soy milk and let sit for 5 minutes until it has thickened then add bananas and purée with stick blender.

In a small pan over low heat, sauté cherries, gently mashing them to release juices.

Add water, cane sugar, a pinch of cinnamon and nutmeg, and cornstarch to thicken. Reduce for 3–4 minutes.

Preheat non-stick pan over medium heat with 1 tbsp oil.

Soak the bread slices in banana and flax mixture flipping each side so it is generously coated. Hold bread above the mixture to allow excess to drip off. Fry in skillet for 2–3 minutes on each side. You will need to add more oil to the pan as you go along.

Layer peaches and cherry compote on top of French toast and bon appétit.

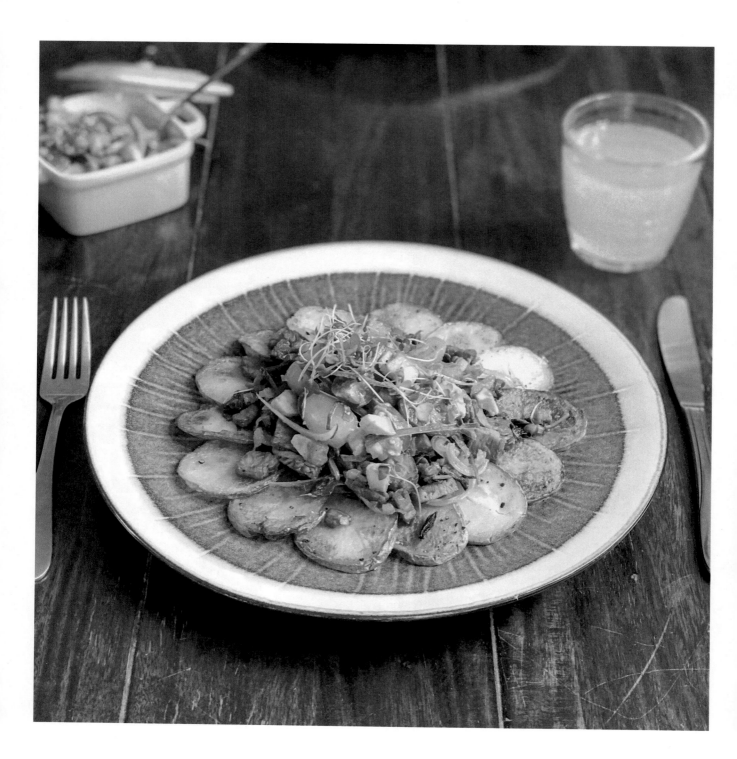

Patatas Bravas with Tempeh
&
Roasted Garlic Kale

This is our take on a dish we saw a lot of while travelling in Spain with River. Although sometimes served with fish or chorizo and a variety of sauces, we've put a plant-based finish on ours. Using "garlicy" kale, smoky tempeh, and then topped with an avocado and grape tomato salsa, the flavours and textures of the dish really allowed us to take a favourite and make it our own plant-based version. The crispy potato also allowed us to pull the wool over River's eyes as he called them French fries, loving the crunch and crispiness of the potatoes.

Ready in 30 minutes   Serves 2

2 redskin potatoes, sliced ⅛ inch thick
4 tbsp avocado oil
¼ white onion, thinly sliced
3 oz bacon tempeh
1 clove garlic, minced
1 small handful of baby kale or chopped kale
broccoli sprouts for garnish (optional)

Tomato Avocado Salsa

12 grape tomatoes sliced in quarters
1 avocado, diced small
¼ red onion, diced small
1 clove garlic
1 tbsp lime juice
2 tbsp cilantro, chopped (optional)
sea salt and pepper to taste

In a large cast iron skillet, heat 4 tbsp of oil over medium heat.

Layer potato slices flat around the base of the skillet and season the potatoes. Fry potatoes for 4–5 minutes on each side until they become brown and crispy. Remove potatoes from skillet; pat dry with paper towel to remove excess oil.

Repeat the above step if you need more potatoes.

While potatoes are cooking, prepare tomato avocado salsa. Combine tomatoes, avocado, red onion, garlic, lime juice, and cilantro and season with sea salt and pepper. Stir until all ingredients are well combined. Salsa makes 6 servings.

Sauté onions, garlic, and tempeh for 3 minutes until onions become light brown and translucent. Add kale until it wilts and remove from heat.

Layer potatoes around the base of a plate. Add tempeh, kale, and onions. Top with tomato avocado salsa and broccoli sprouts, and serve. This makes a great shared plate.

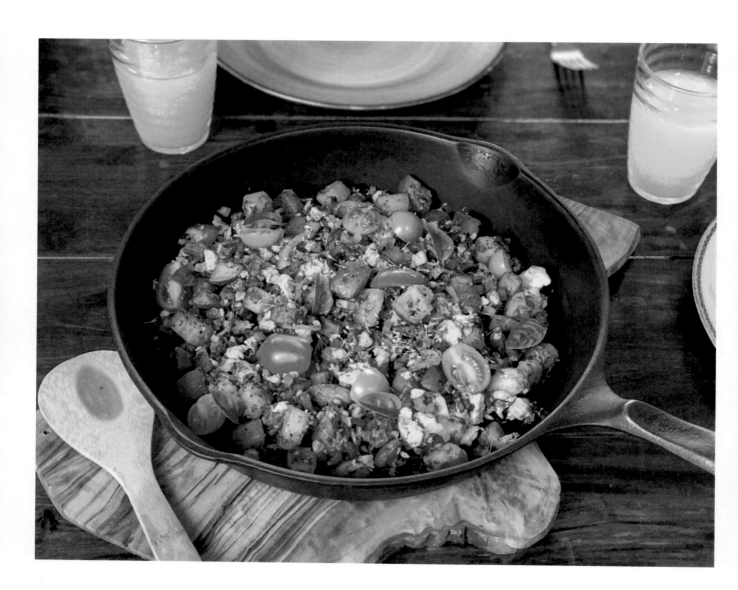

"Bacon & Egg" Skillet

This hash works perfect for a small family breakfast or even large gatherings of friends and family. As soon as this dish starts coming together in the pan or skillet, the household begins to wake up with the amazing aromatics from the spices, vegetables, and herbs. The tempeh adds a beautiful flavour and crunch of crispy bacon and it takes most by surprise when we reveal it's 100% plant-based.

Ready in 30 minutes   Serves 4

4 medium redskin potatoes, diced
¼ onion, diced
5 mushrooms, sliced
½ red pepper, diced small
⅓ pk bacon tempeh
½ tsp smoked paprika
¼ tsp thyme
1 clove garlic, minced
1 tbsp + 1 tsp of oil
fresh basil for garnish (optional)
sea salt and pepper to taste

Egg Mix
175 g firm tofu
1 tbsp nutritional yeast
1 tsp onion powder
1 tsp turmeric
sea salt and pepper to taste

In a large skillet, heat oil over medium heat. Add potatoes, thyme, smoked paprika, sea salt, and pepper. Sauté for 8–10 minutes. While potatoes are sautéing prepare egg mix.

Crumble tofu into a medium bowl; add nutritional yeast, onion powder, turmeric, sea salt, and pepper; and stir until well mixed.

Next, add onions, red pepper, mushrooms, and garlic. Sauté for 6-8 minutes until potatoes are cooked. Add tofu egg mix and crumble tempeh into the skillet. Sauté for 2-3 minutes. Garnish with basil and serve.

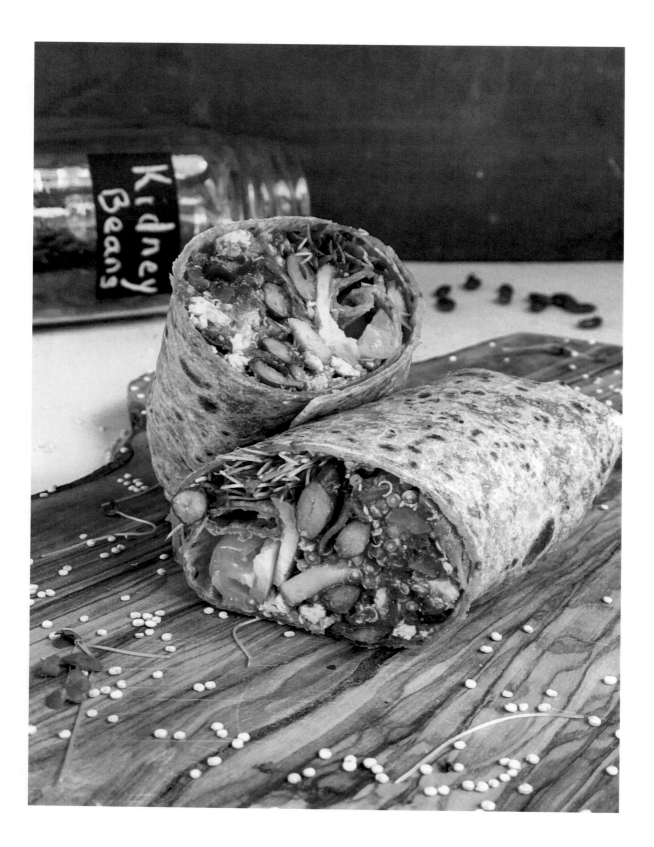

Breakfast Burrito

A quick egg sandwich or wrap is a classic go to for our morning breakfast, and the ease of wrapping it up and taking it to work is another bonus. This wrap has a southwestern feel and with all the flavours going on it's hard to tell it's not really scrambled eggs inside.

Gluten-free   Ready in 30-35 minutes   Serves 6

1 (15 oz) kidney beans or ¾ cup dry kidney beans cook, strain, and rinse (see chart on page xix)
½ cup quinoa, dry
½ red pepper, julienne
½ white onion, julienne
8 small mushrooms, sliced
1 tbsp avocado oil
1 cup vegetable stock or water
1 cup canned tomatoes
2 cloves garlic, minced
2 tsp chili powder
½ tsp cumin
¼ tsp coriander
½ tsp smoked paprika
¼ tsp crushed chili (optional)
sea salt and pepper to taste
1 medium tomato, diced
1 avocado, diced
broccoli sprouts (optional)
6 (10") tortilla wraps, gluten-free

Egg Mix
175 g firm tofu
1 tbsp nutritional yeast
1 tsp onion powder
1 tsp turmeric
sea salt and pepper to taste

In a medium pot, cook quinoa in vegetable stock or water and set aside. See chart on page xix.

Prepare egg mix. Crumble tofu into a medium bowl; add nutritional yeast, onion powder, turmeric, salt, and pepper; and stir until well mixed.

In a large skillet, heat oil over medium heat. Sauté onions, mushrooms, and red pepper; season with sea salt and pepper for 5 minutes.

Add garlic, chili powder, cumin, coriander, smoked paprika, and crushed chilies and sauté for 3 minutes.

Add the tomatoes and kidney beans. Reduce until most of the liquid is absorbed.

Add quinoa and tofu egg mix and stir together. Cook for 2-3 minutes.

Place a tortilla wrap on a flat surface. Take ¾ of a cup of the filling and spread out in the centre of the tortilla. Layer tomato, avocado, and broccoli sprouts on top. Wrap them up folding in the ends as you go. Cut and serve.

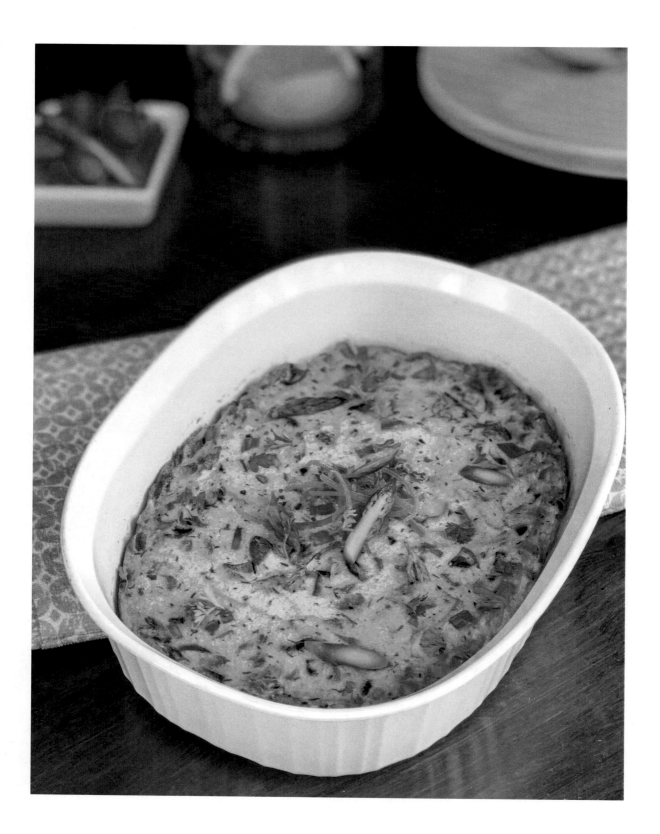

"You Gotta Try This" Frittata

When transitioning to a plant-based diet, we found that many breakfast meals usually consisted of some sort of "bacon and eggs" dish. That didn't leave much choice for hearty morning meals. Good thing that's not true. Taking time to tweak the textures, flavours, and the look of the tofu that we use in place of eggs really helped us develop something that looks and tastes just like a frittata.

We often forget the benefits of having nutritious and healthy starts to our days. We hear over and over that breakfast is the most important meal but we can overlook it and tend to forget that this is our morning kick start. Growing together as a family we now fully understand the importance of eating right in the morning, and this is one of those dishes that has us feeling amazing. Eat great, feel great, do great!

Gluten-free   Ready in 40 minutes   Serves 4

¼ large onion, diced
½ cup asparagus, finely diced
1 cup mushrooms, diced
1 tbsp avocado oil
½ tsp garlic powder
½ tsp onion powder
1 tsp thyme
1 tsp smoked paprika
1 ½ tsp blackstrap molasses
350g medium tofu
2 tbsp nutritional yeast
1 tsp turmeric
1 tbsp lemon juice
sea salt and pepper to taste
fresh parsley, chopped for garnish (optional)

Preheat oven to 350°F. Lightly grease a pie plate.

In a medium mixing bowl, add asparagus, mushrooms, and onions. Add avocado oil, smoked paprika, thyme, onion powder, garlic powder, blackstrap molasses, sea salt, and pepper. Mix.

Line a baking sheet with parchment paper and spread the vegetables on the baking sheet. Bake for 8-10 minutes.

While vegetables are roasting prepare the tofu "eggs". In a medium bowl add tofu, nutritional yeast, turmeric, lemon juice, sea salt, and pepper. With a stick blender, purée everything together.

Once the vegetables are done, remove from the oven and mix into the tofu "egg" mix. Stir together and pour into the pie plate.

Bake for 20-25 minutes. Remove from oven and let rest for 2-3 minutes before cutting and serving.

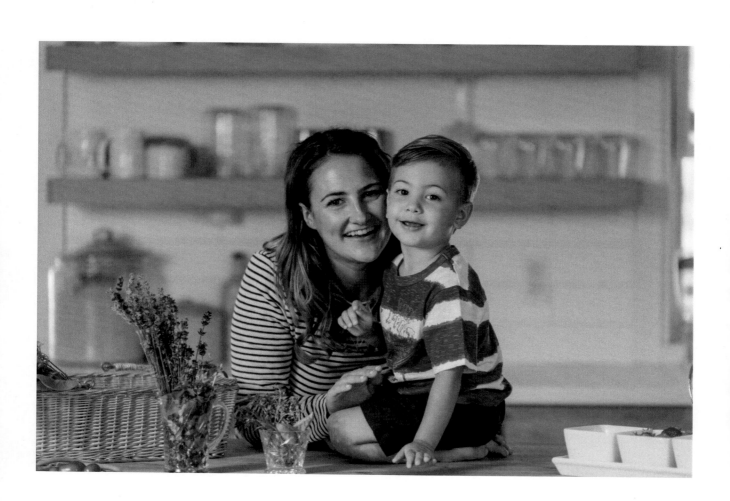

SAVOURY
SIDES

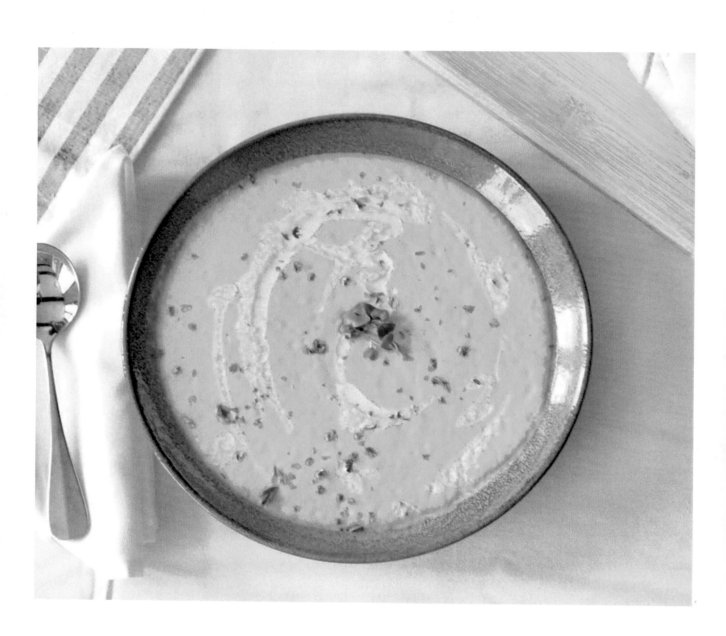

Ginger & Miso Squash Soup

The many nurturing, feel-good ingredients in this recipe turn a simple fall squash soup into a year-round favourite. Squash has always been a part of our diet and when fall rolls around it's easy to find so many uses for it. When River was a baby, we made sure to roast extra and create a simple squash purée that we could freeze in ice cubes for meals throughout the month.

Gluten-free   Ready in 1 hour   Makes 12 cups

4 cups roasted squash
4 cups vegetable stock
1 (400 ml) can coconut milk
2 small apples, peeled and chopped
½ medium onion, chopped
2 tbsp extra virgin olive oil
2 cloves garlic, minced
1 tbsp fresh ginger, minced
⅛ tsp each turmeric, cinnamon, star anise
   Use 2 whole pcs of star anise in place of
   ground, if needed
1 bay leaf
pinch of ground dried clove
1 tbsp miso paste, gluten-free
sea salt and pepper to taste

Preheat oven to 350°F. Peel and dice squash; toss with 1 tbsp oil, sea salt, and pepper; then put on a baking sheet and roast until soft: approximately 15 minutes. Do not allow the squash to become darkened as it will discolour the soup. A little browning on the edges is OK as it gives extra flavour.

As the squash is roasting, in a large pot heat the other tbsp of oil over medium heat. Add onions and apples and sauté for approximately 12 minutes.

Add garlic and ginger and sauté for another 3 minutes.

By now the squash should be roasted. Add squash to the pot with the spices and sauté for 3 minutes. Add the vegetable stock and simmer for 20 minutes. Remove star anise pieces and bay leaf before you purée with stick blender. Add the coconut milk and miso paste and purée again. Check seasoning and serve.

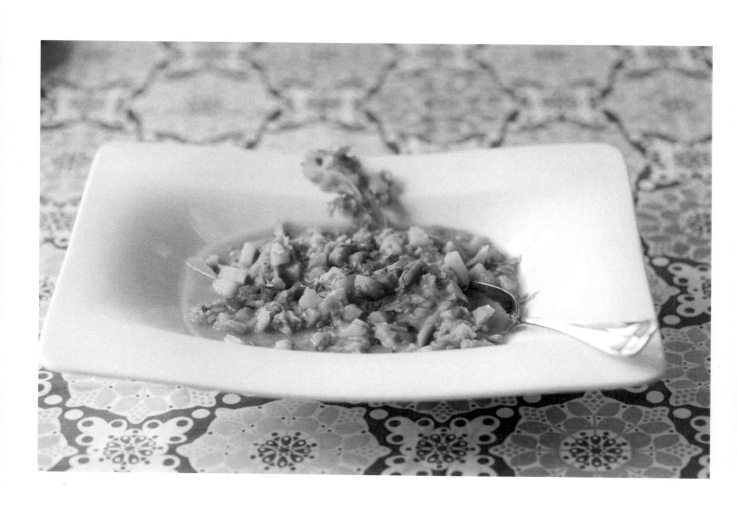

Save Yourself Some Thyme
Split Pea Soup

Split pea soup was a favourite growing up, particularly once the weather turned cold. If you want to save yourself some time, place all ingredients into a crockpot and let simmer until split peas are cooked. Here is another great example of a meal that can be easily puréed into baby food. This soup provides a good source of iron, especially if you leave the skins on the potatoes.

Gluten-free   Ready in 1 hour 15 minutes   Makes 12 cups

2 medium potatoes, washed and diced with skins on
3 carrots, peeled and diced
1 medium onion, diced
3 stalks celery, diced
1 cup split peas
1 tbsp extra virgin olive oil
10 ½ cups vegetable stock
2 cloves garlic, minced
5-6 sprigs of fresh thyme or 2 tsp dried
2 bay leaves
sea salt and pepper to taste

In a large pot, heat oil over medium heat.

Sauté carrots, onions, and celery for about 5 minutes or until onions become translucent. Then add in garlic, quickly sauté, and add stock.

Add potatoes, split peas, thyme, and bay leaves. Cover and let simmer for 60 minutes (until peas are cooked). Add sea salt and pepper to taste and serve.

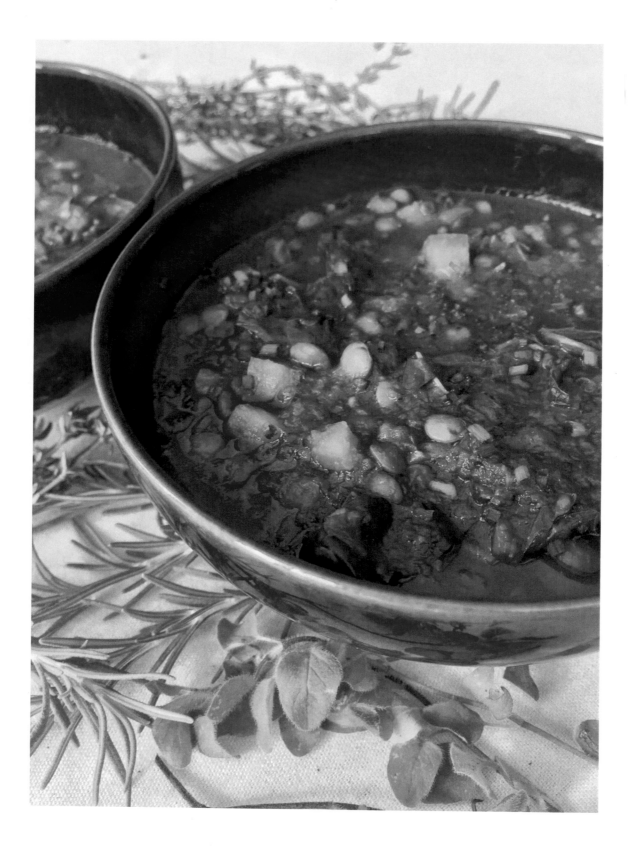

Tomato, Kale, & Lentil Soup

This is a stick to your ribs kind of soup. The lentils add a nice density and using black beans or beluga lentils also works well. We like to garnish with fresh diced tomato and parsley, and serve with warm bread.

Gluten-free   Ready in 35 minutes   Makes 10 cups

1 (28 oz) can tomatoes
4 cups kale
1 medium onion, diced
3 stalks celery, diced
2 cups green lentils, dry
2 tsp Italian seasoning
1 tsp dried parsley
2 cloves garlic, minced
3 bay leaves
6 cups vegetable stock
1 tbsp extra virgin olive oil
sea salt and pepper to taste

In a large pot, heat oil over medium heat. Add onions and celery, and season with sea salt and pepper. Sauté for 5 minutes. Add garlic and continue to sauté for 2 more minutes.

Add tomatoes and vegetable stock, and purée with a stick blender.

Add dry lentils, bay leaves, and Italian seasoning. Simmer for 20 minutes then add kale. Continue to cook for 2 more minutes. Check seasoning and serve.

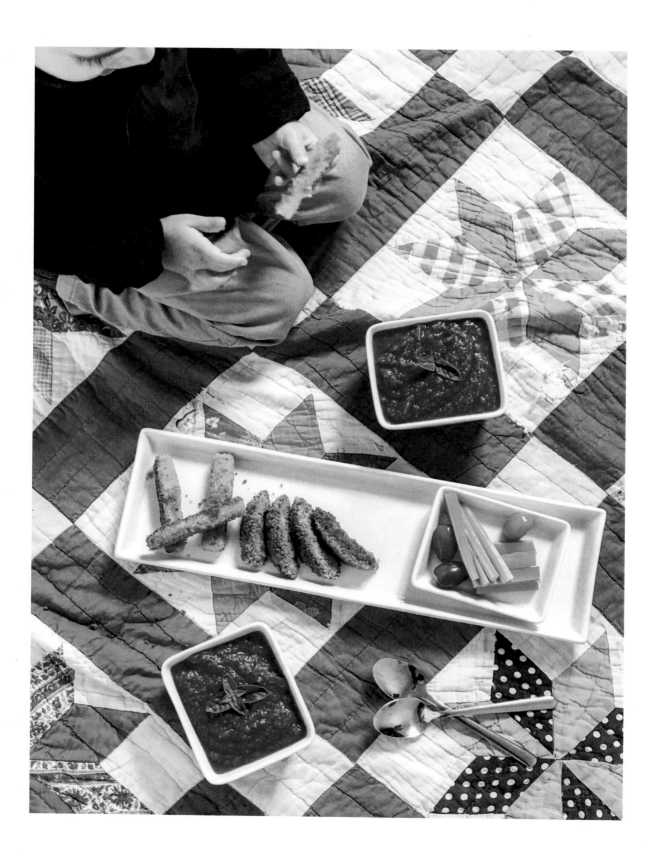

Charred Tomato Soup with Avocado & Zucchini Fries

Tomato soup was a childhood favourite. We had to include this one, not just for River but for us! We love the smoky charred flavours of this soup and dipping the avocado and zucchini into the tomato goodness just makes it a perfect and fun match. The Charred Tomato Soup is gluten-free but not the Avocado and Zucchini fries.

Ready in 1 hour   Makes 8 cups

2 (28 oz cans) diced tomatoes
1 medium onion, diced
½ cup carrots, peeled and diced
3 stalks celery, diced
4 cloves garlic
1 tbsp fresh thyme or oregano
1 tbsp smoked paprika
1 cup vegetable stock
¼ cup fresh basil, chopped
2 tbsp avocado oil or extra virgin olive oil
1 tsp sugar
sea salt and pepper to taste

Avocado and Zucchini Fries

1 small zucchini
1 medium avocado
1 cup panko bread crumbs
⅓ cup flour
1 cup soy milk + 2 tbsp flax meal
¼ cup oil for frying

Preheat oven to broil. Line baking sheet with parchment paper.

Drain the cans of tomatoes and set the liquid aside. Toss the onions, celery, carrots, and garlic in 1 tbsp oil, season with sea salt and pepper, and spread on baking sheet with the drained tomatoes. Place in the oven until the vegetables are soft and the tomatoes begin to blacken and char (don't worry if they look burnt as it will add more flavour) about 30 minutes.

Heat a large pot over medium heat with 1 tbsp of oil. Transfer the charred vegetables to the pot and add the smoked paprika and fresh thyme. Continue sautéing for 3 minutes, then add the tomatoes, strained tomato juice, vegetable stock, sugar, and basil. Bring to a boil and reduce to simmer for 20 minutes. Remove from heat and purée and season.

For the avocado and zucchini fries, cut the avocado in half, removing the pit. Cut the avocado into 12 wedges and set aside for breading. Cut the zucchini fries into 3 inch by ¼ inch batons and set aside for breading.

We recommend breading the zucchini first and then the avocado. Start by placing the flour, milk/flax mixture, and bread crumbs each in their own medium bowl. Dredge the zucchini in the flour and then into the milk/flax mixture. Once coated, finish by gently breading with the bread crumbs. Try keeping one hand dry for flour and bread crumbs, and the other hand wet for the milk/flax mixture; it creates less mess. Place finished zucchini fries onto plate to reserve for frying. Repeat for avocado fries.

To prepare the avocado and zucchini fries, begin by heating a medium frying pan with 2 tbsp of oil over medium heat. Once oil is heated, add the fries 4-5 at a time and fry for 2-3 minutes on each side until golden brown. Remove from pan and repeat with the remaining fries. Add more oil for frying if needed. You want a nice crispy brown coating on the outside. Serve along with the soup.

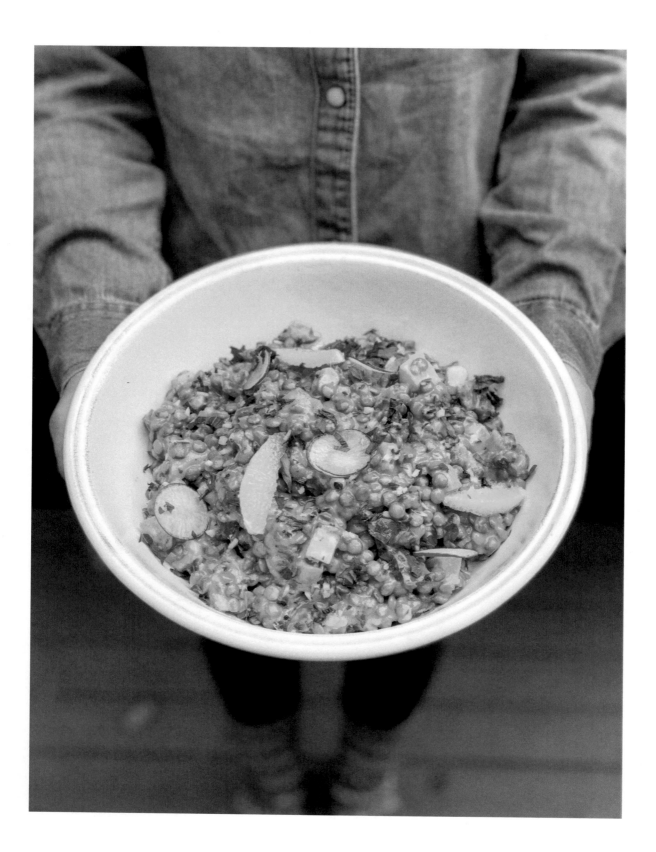

Fall Squash & Lentil Salad

This is our favourite salad to take on picnics or to BBQs in late summer or early autumn. Bright fall colours let us know the season's harvest is just around the corner.

Gluten-free   Ready in 35 minutes   Serves 8

2 cups green lentils, dry
2 cups butternut or kabocha squash,
**   medium diced**
1 cup red pepper, medium diced
1 cup zucchini, medium diced
2 tbsp avocado oil
sea salt and pepper to taste

Citrus Flax Vinaigrette

2 tbsp maple syrup
2 tbsp Dijon mustard
2 tbsp apple cider vinegar
½ orange, juiced and zested
1 cup avocado oil or canola oil
1 tsp fresh ginger, minced
2 tbsp parsley, chopped
¼ tsp flax meal

Preheat oven to 350°F. Line two baking sheets with parchment paper.

Rinse lentils and cook (see chart on page xix). Remove from heat, rinse, and strain off water. Place lentils in fridge to cool down.

Peel and dice squash; toss squash in 1 tbsp of oil, sea salt, and pepper. Spread on baking sheet and roast for 15-20 minutes, until lightly browned and softened. Remove from oven and cool.

Toss red pepper and zucchini with additional tbsp oil, sea salt, and pepper and roast on a separate baking sheet for 8-12 minutes. Remove from oven and cool.

For the vinaigrette: In a medium bowl combine Dijon, maple syrup, orange juice and zest, apple cider vinegar, ginger, flax meal, and parsley and whisk well. Slowly add the oil while whisking vigorously until mixture and oil lightly emulsify. Season with sea salt and pepper as needed.

Combine the lentils, roasted squash, zucchini, pepper, and vinaigrette and gently mix. Voila!

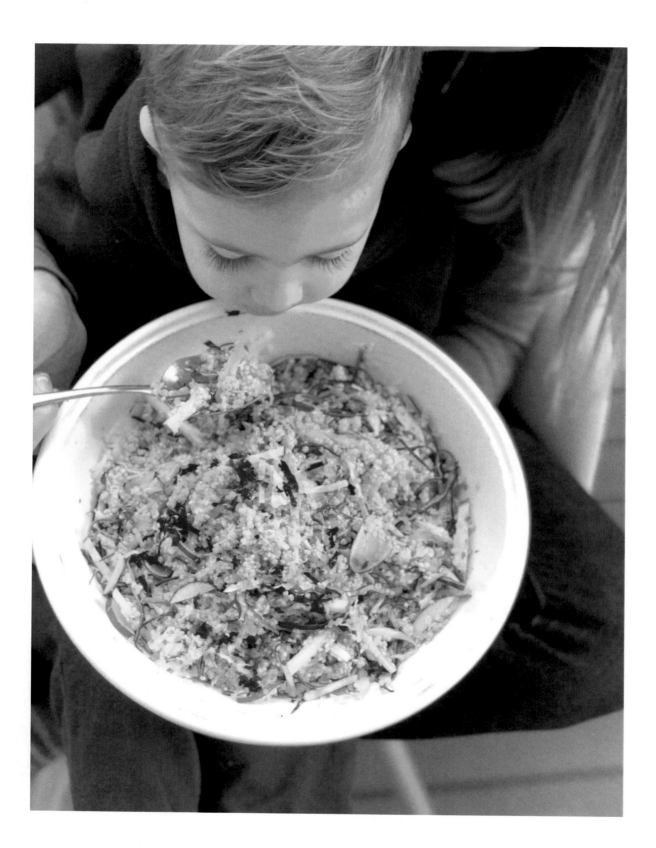

Rainbow Radish, Apple, & Quinoa Salad

Another in-a-pinch salad that is quick, easy, and refreshing with the citrus-ginger notes. In the summer heat, we love sitting on the deck for meals or snacks. These light salads make for a perfect mid-afternoon bite or alongside any meal.

Gluten-free   Ready in 25 minutes   Serves 4

1 cup quinoa, dry
½ cup radish, sliced
¾ cup savoy cabbage, shredded
¾ cup purple cabbage, shredded
1 Granny Smith apple, peeled, and sliced
  into matchsticks

Lime-Ginger Dressing

1 lime, juiced
½-¾ lime zest
2 tsp fresh ginger, grated
⅓ cup avocado oil
1 tsp maple syrup (optional)
sea salt and pepper to taste

Cook quinoa (see chart on page xix). Place in the fridge to cool and prevent from overcooking.

To make dressing, whisk together lime juice, zest, ginger, oil, maple syrup, and sea salt and pepper.

Once quinoa has cooled, combine all the ingredients in a medium mixing bowl and toss gently with the dressing. Serve and enjoy.

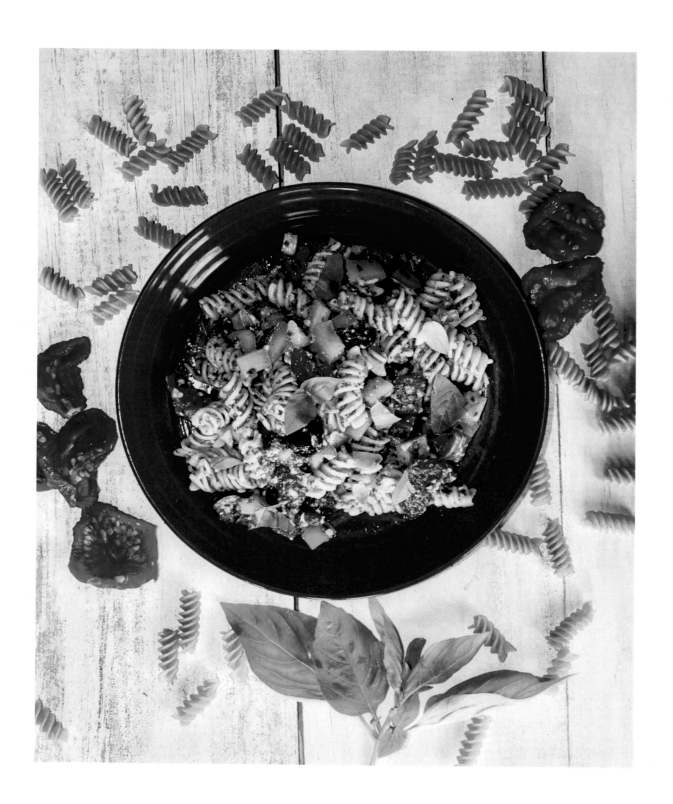

Garden Basil Pesto Pasta with Sun-Dried Tomatoes & Olives

Getting dirty in the garden is one of River's favourite things to do in the spring as we begin planting new herbs and vegetables. Being able to make pesto and add herbs to all our dishes is a bonus. This creamy pesto is sweet, nutty, and full of citrus notes, pairing perfectly with the salty olives and sun-dried tomato. To make this dish gluten-free just substitute regular pasta for a gluten-free option.

Ready in 25 minutes   Serves 4

2 cups fusilli pasta
½ cup Kalamata or green olives, cut in half
½ cup sundried tomatoes, chopped
1 yellow pepper, small diced
½ red onion, small diced
1 cup pesto

Pesto

½ cup walnuts
1 ⅓ cups basil
1 small clove garlic, minced
½ lemon, juiced
1 tbsp nutritional yeast
½ cup olive oil
sea salt and pepper to taste

Bring a medium pot of salted water to a boil and cook pasta as per directions on box.

In a mini chopper or high power blender, add walnuts, basil, garlic, lemon juice, nutritional yeast, olive oil, and sea salt and pepper to taste and purée.

In a medium bowl, mix pasta, veggies, and pesto sauce. Check seasoning and serve.

Tip

When cooking pasta always salt the water; it will bring out the flavour. Many people add oil to the water when cooking pasta, but if you have the time there is no need to; some say it does more harm than good. Gently stir your pasta as it is added to the boiling water, and every so often repeat; this will help break up the starches in the pasta, thereby preventing the noodles from clinging to each other.

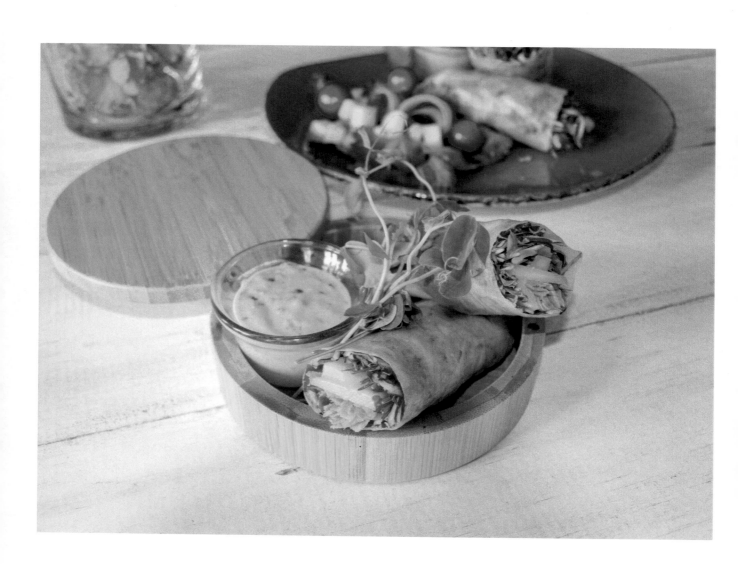

Rice Paper Spring Rolls with Coconut Peanut Sauce

These are great to have when out on light adventures with the family. We quickly pack them in a small Tupperware container and they're a nice and easy snack to have anywhere we stop. We also like adding leaf lettuce, peppers or basil leaves, or even crisp apple and peach to replace the mango when in season.

Gluten-free   Ready in 15-20 minutes   Makes 6 Rolls

¾ cup cucumber
30 g pea shoots
¾ cup carrot
¾ cup mango
1 ½ cup purple cabbage
6 tsp cilantro
6 rice paper wraps 10 g/wrap

Coconut Peanut Sauce
¼ cup coconut milk
¼ cup peanut butter
juice of ½ lime
1 ½ tsp turbinado sugar
1 cloves of garlic, minced
2 tsp fresh ginger, minced
sea salt and pepper
2 tbsp cilantro, chopped
2 tbsp sesame oil
Yields ¾ cup sauce

Begin by preparing the coconut peanut sauce. In a small saucepan on low heat, add the coconut milk, peanut butter, and sugar. Whisk together allowing the sugar to dissolve. Place all ingredients in a mini chop or blender and purée.

Julienne cucumber, carrots, and mango into 3-inch-long match sticks and shred the cabbage. Set each vegetable aside as you get ready to roll your spring rolls.

Run rice paper wraps under water for 5 seconds. You don't want them to be soft or you will have trouble rolling them.

Lay the wraps on a flat surface and start building your spring rolls. Add cabbage, cucumber, mango, carrots, pea shoots, and cilantro. Roll them up folding in the ends as you go. Try not to overfill as they will be harder to roll. Cut spring rolls in half before serving with the coconut peanut sauce. One serving equals one roll.

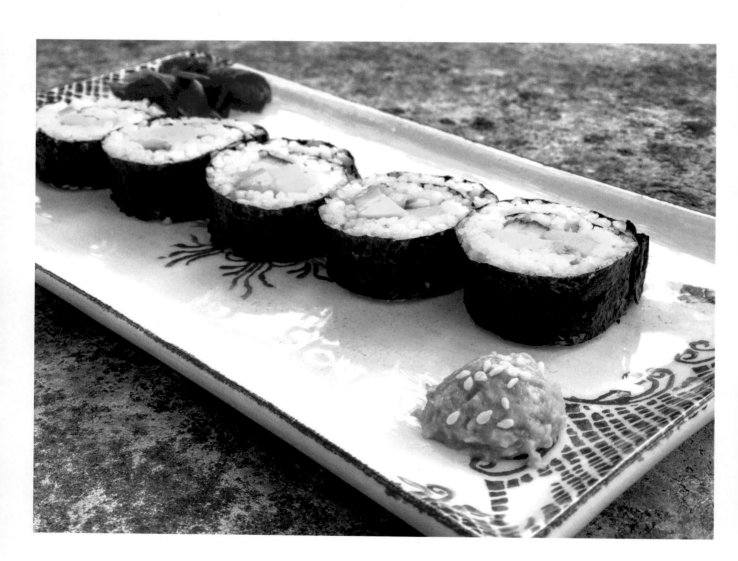

Avocado Sushi Roll

We didn't grow up eating sushi—or even thinking about it as young children—but as we grew older and began dining out we always had sushi nights. As we witness the impact we are having on our oceans, we created plant-based sushi recipes and ideas. We like keeping sushi in our meal planning as the nori is a good source of iodine. We will often substitute mangoes for local peaches, and we found River enjoys the textures of the rice and sweetness of the fruit.

Gluten-free   Ready in 25 minutes   Makes 5 rolls

2 cups sushi rice
2 cups water
2 tbsp rice vinegar
2 tbsp agave nectar
nori sheets
½ cucumber, matchstick slices
½ mango or peach, matchstick slices
1 avocado, matchstick slices

Rinse and strain sushi rice.

In a medium pot, add water to rice and cook (see chart on page xix).

Turn off the stove. Add rice vinegar and agave; stir until well mixed. Cover and set aside for 5 minutes.

Remove cover and allow to cool for another 5 minutes.

Lay a nori sheet on a flat surface and spread out rice evenly on the sheet. Leave 1 inch not covered in rice at the bottom of the nori sheet.

½ inch down from the top of the sushi sheet start layering your avocado, cucumber, and mango or peaches horizontally across the sheet.

Roll beginning at the top. Cut into medallions and serve. One serving equals one roll.

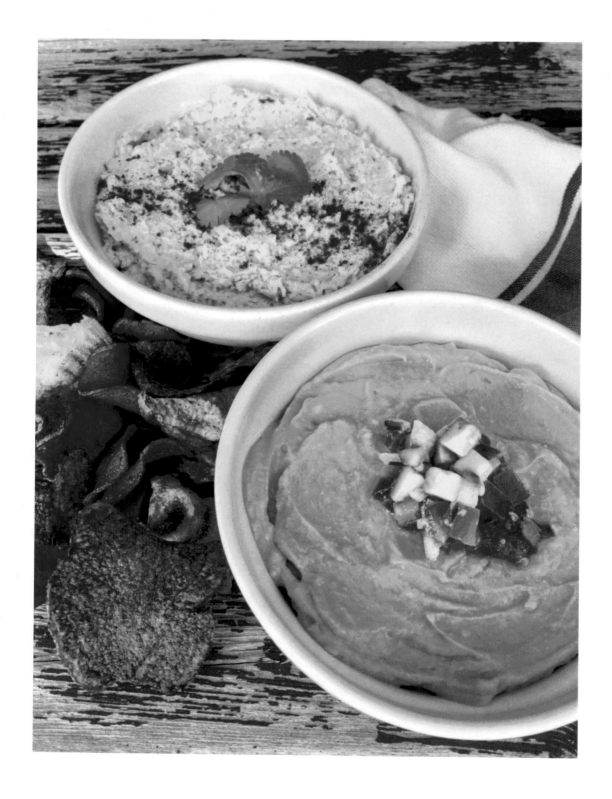

Lemon Cumin Hummus & Citrus Guacamole

Finding healthy snacks can be challenging. Having quick dips or spreads on hand for vegetable crudité, tortilla chips, or crackers to dip in, is ideal. They make for a nice interactive snack for larger parties, too. These are both quick, healthy, and perfect for dipping. I prefer using the stick blender to purée, as it reduces the mess, but you can use a food processor as well.

Gluten-free   Ready 10-15 minutes   Serves 6

Hummus

1 (15 oz) can chickpeas or ¾ cup dry chick-peas, cook, strain and rinse (see chart on page xix)
1 lemon, juiced
2 cloves garlic, minced
¼ cup extra virgin olive oil
¼ cup tahini
3 tbsp canola oil
¾ tsp cumin
¼ cup cilantro, minced (optional)
sea salt and pepper to taste

Guacamole

2 avocados
1 lime, juiced
1 large clove garlic, minced
½ red pepper, diced
½ medium tomato
¼ tsp cumin
2 tbsp fresh cilantro, minced
sea salt and pepper to taste

Hummus

Drain and rinse the chickpeas. Reserve the liquid from the canned chickpeas for aiolis or for other egg replacers.

Place all ingredients together in a large bowl. With a stick blender, purée and serve.

Guacamole

Place all ingredients in a bowl. With a stick blender, purée and serve.

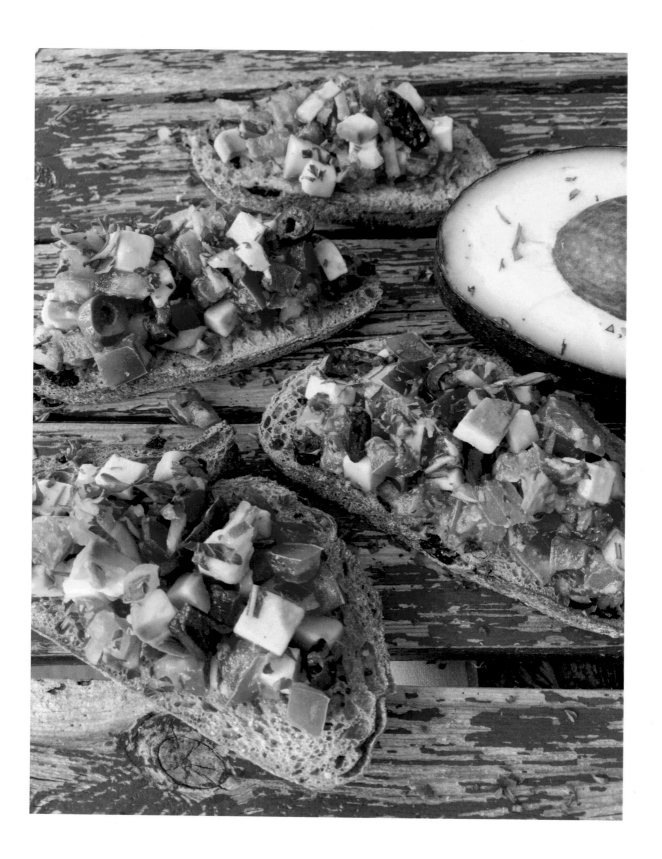

Heirloom Tomato & Avocado Bruschetta

My all time favourite. We love doing theme nights for dinner, like tapas night or pub night and doing a few smaller snack items instead of one large meal. We always include a version of bruschetta. It was on one of these nights when we started the joke that, when River is older, all his friends are going to ask their parents if they can eat dinner at our house because we are always cooking up delicious meals and snacks. The Bruschetta works just as well if served cold instead of warming in the oven, and try changing the bread and crostini it's served with.

Ready in 20 minutes   Makes 15 pieces

1 loaf French bread, sliced
2 medium tomatoes, finely diced
½ medium red onion, finely diced
½ bell pepper, finely diced
10 black olives, pitted and finely chopped
1 avocado, pitted and small diced
1 clove garlic, minced
3 tbsp fresh basil, chopped
1 tbsp extra virgin olive oil and a little extra
   for drizzling over the bread
1 tsp apple cider vinegar
sea salt and pepper to taste

Preheat the oven to 375°F.

In a large bowl, combine tomatoes, red onion, bell peppers, black olives, avocado, garlic, basil, olive oil, vinegar, and sea salt and pepper to taste.

Place bread on a baking sheet and drizzle olive oil over it. Bake for 5 minutes until lightly brown.

Scoop bruschetta mixture onto bread and place back in the oven for 2 minutes. Remove from oven and serve. One serving equals one piece.

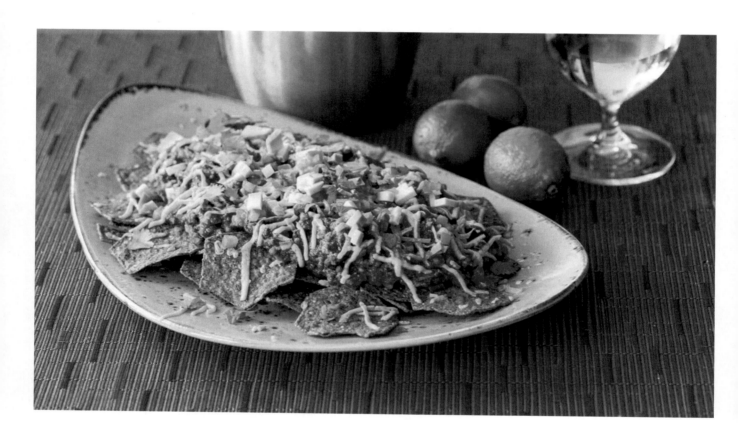

Nachos by Nature

This is another great way to keep some recipes exciting the second night over, and it is a hearty snack for all. We love adding avocado and fresh heirloom tomato whenever we can. Olives and peppers also complement this fun snack.

Gluten-free   Ready in 15 minutes   Serves 4

1/2 bag tortilla chips, gluten-free
2 cups Cool Beans Chili (see recipe on page 65)
½ avocado, small diced
½ tomato, small diced
¾ cup vegan cheese (optional)

Preheat oven to 350°F.

Line a baking sheet with parchment paper and cover it with tortilla chips.

Gently layer Cool Beans Chili over the chips. Top with vegan cheese (optional) and diced avocado and tomato.

Bake for 8-10 minutes. Remove from oven and dig in.

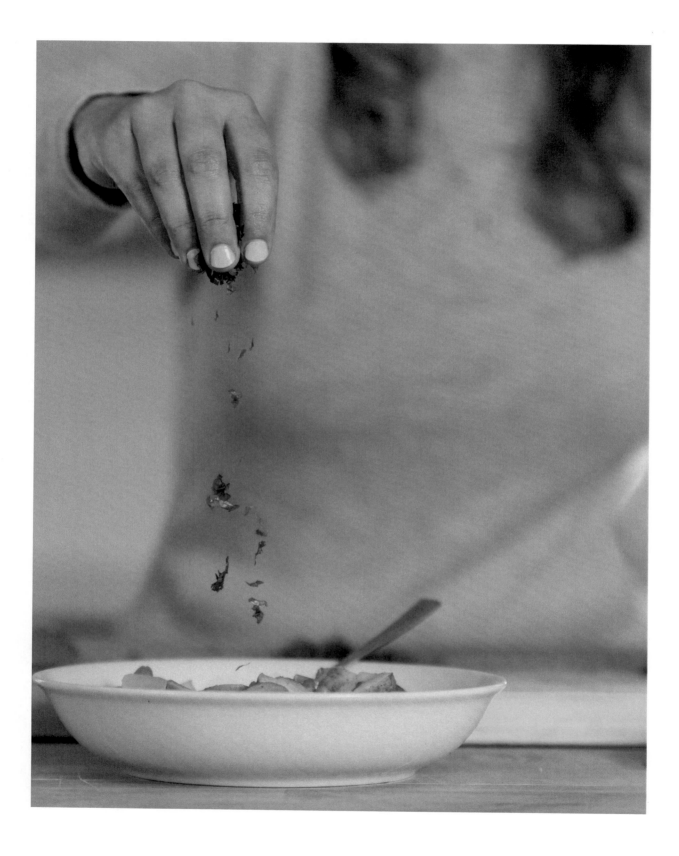

PEACEFUL

PLATES

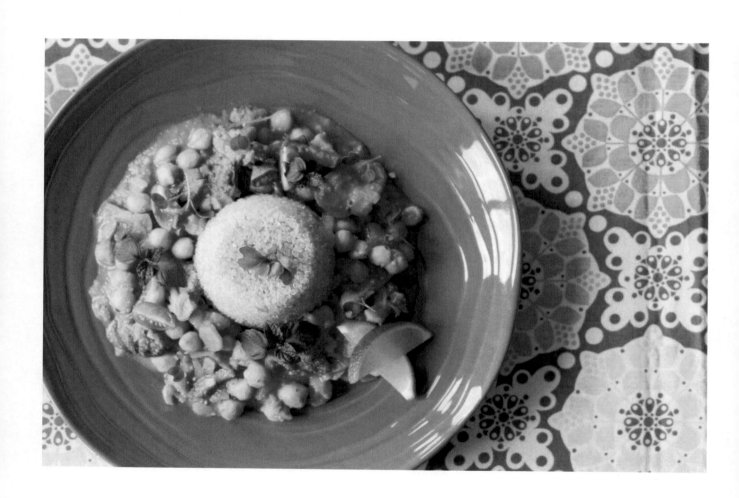

Coconut, Chickpea, & Vegetable Curry with Quinoa

To make life easier in the colder months, it's nice to have those one or two pot dishes that keep you warm on the inside, but also allow you to do it with relative ease. This is one of those dishes. Another bonus is it tastes even better the next day, and though great with the quinoa, using rice and adding warm naan also pairs well and changes it up if using for lunch or dinner the following day.

Gluten-free   Ready in 35 minutes   Serves 6

1 heaping cup butternut squash, peeled and small diced
1 (15 oz) can chickpeas or ¾ of dry chickpeas, cook, strain, and rinse (see chart on page xix)
1 medium onion, small diced
3 small carrots, peeled and diced
½ red bell pepper, small diced
4 mushrooms, sliced or quartered
1 stalk celery, small diced
2 cups frozen or fresh broccoli florets
1 cup quinoa, dry
1 (400 ml) can coconut milk
1 tbsp coconut oil
½ tbsp ginger, minced
2 cloves garlic, minced
2 tbsp curry powder
2 tbsp red curry paste
sea salt and pepper to taste

For how to cook quinoa see chart on page xix.

You can either boil the squash or roast it in the oven. Once cooked, set aside.

In a large saucepan, heat oil over medium heat.

Add onions, carrots, red pepper, mushrooms, celery, sea salt, and pepper, and sauté for 5 minutes. Add broccoli, ginger, garlic, curry powder, and red curry paste, and continue to sauté until onions are translucent. If the spices start sticking to the pan add a little water.

In a medium bowl, add squash and coconut milk and purée with a stick blender. Pour into saucepan with veggies and spices.

Add chickpeas and let simmer for 5 minutes.

Place in serving dish and serve over warm quinoa.

Tip
You can also substitute 1 cup of canned tomatoes for squash. We like using either butternut squash or Cucurbita squash.

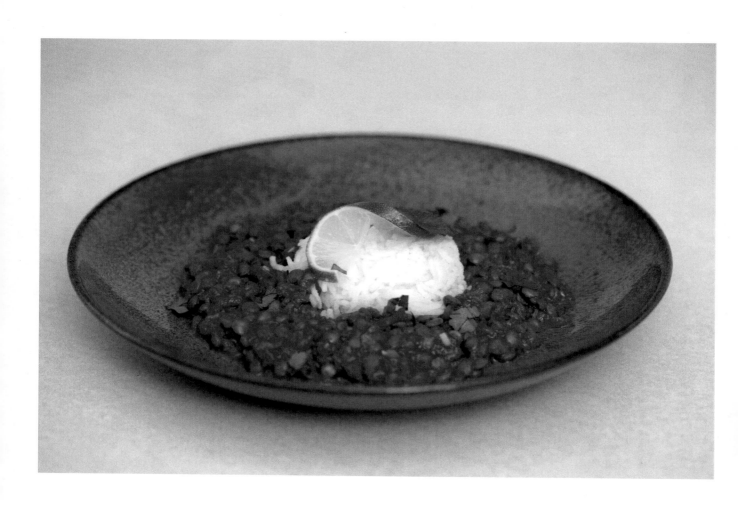

Not so Dull, Dhal

Our love for Indian cuisine has grown stronger over the years. It is another culture of food that always seems to have more than one vegetarian option on the menu when dining out or picking up. Even before becoming plant-based, we found ourselves ordering the vegetable curries, spinach paneer, or a variation of vegetable dahl, or eggplant and cauliflower korma. We introduced these spices and flavours early on with River and found this dish is a family favourite.

Gluten-free   Ready in 30 minutes   Serves 8

1 ½ cups basmati rice, dry
2 cups green lentils, dry
1 medium onion, diced
1 (28 oz) can diced tomatoes
6.75 oz coconut milk
3 cloves garlic, minced
1 tbsp ginger, grated
1-2 tbsp coconut oil
2 tbsp red curry paste
2 tbsp curry powder
sea salt and pepper to taste

In a medium pot, cook basmati rice (see chart on page xix).

In a medium pot, cook lentils (see chart on page xix). Strain and rinse with cool water.

In a large saucepan, heat oil over medium heat. Sauté onions for 5 minutes, add ginger and garlic, and continue to sauté for another couple of minutes.

Add curry powder and paste and stir. Add a can of diced tomatoes, coconut milk, and cooked lentils.

Let simmer for 5 minutes and add salt and pepper to taste. Serve over rice and enjoy!

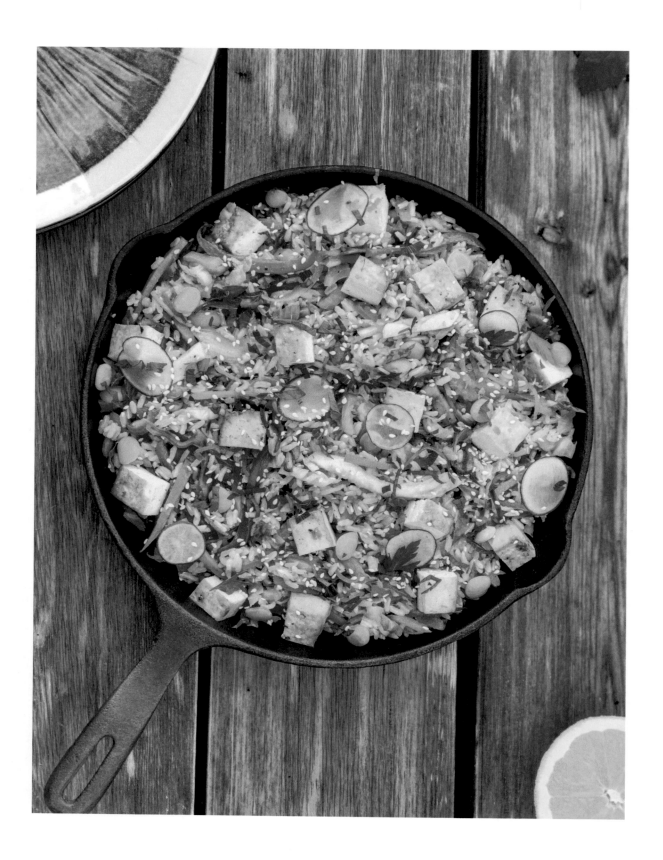

Miso & Orange Crispy Asian Tofu Stir Fry

Fried rice started out as an easy dish to use up any leftover vegetables or rice we might have hanging around. As we began incorporating tofu into a lot of our dishes we noticed how much better we could flavour it with different marinades and rubs. We developed this fried rice that gives off such bright and warm flavours that we needed to add it to the book. River has always enjoyed fried rice, and this orange ginger marinated dish only adds to that enjoyment. Adding the miso adds not only more taste but it is also beneficial for the probiotics.

Gluten-free   Ready in 40-45 minutes   Serves 4

350 g super firm tofu
1 cup long grain brown rice, dry
1 cup onion, thinly sliced
1 cup carrot, peeled and sliced
½ cup bell peppers, julienned
1 cup edamame beans, out of shell
1 cup mushrooms, sliced or quartered
1 cup purple cabbage, thinly sliced
1 cup green cabbage, thinly sliced
2 tbsp tamari, gluten-free or soy sauce
2 cloves garlic, minced
3 tbsp avocado oil for frying
1 tsp sesame oil for frying
2 tbsp white sesame seeds, toasted
sea salt and pepper to taste

Tofu Marinade

2 tbsp tamari, gluten-free, or soy sauce
2 tbsp maple syrup
1 ½ tbsp rice vinegar
1 clove garlic, minced
1 tsp ginger, minced
1 tbsp miso, gluten-free
1 tsp orange zest
1 tbsp orange juice, fresh

Cook brown rice (see chart on page xix).

Prepare the tofu marinade. Combine all ingredients and whisk together.

Slice and dice veggies. Now rice should be done. Transfer rice into a bowl and let cool in the fridge.

Remove tofu from package a press out excess water. Divide tofu into 4 rectangular slices approximately ½ inch thick and place in marinade. We try and marinate for 2 hours but if pressed for time 10 minutes is fine as we reuse the marinade in the recipe.

In a small frying pan, heat 2 tbsp oil over medium heat.

Remove 4 tbsp of marinade from the tofu (this will be used later when frying the rice). Fry the tofu 3-4 minutes per side, until brown. Deglaze the pan with remaining marinade and remove from heat. Once slightly cooled, dice the tofu into even sized cubes and save for adding into the sir fry.

In a large skillet, heat 1 tbsp oil and 1 tsp sesame oil over medium heat. Add all vegetables except for garlic. Sauté for 4 minutes then add garlic and continue to cook for 3 minutes. Combine the brown rice with soy sauce and 2 tbsp of the marinade, turn off heat, and stir.

Add tofu to rice and pour any leftover marinade over the rice. Stir, plate, and serve.

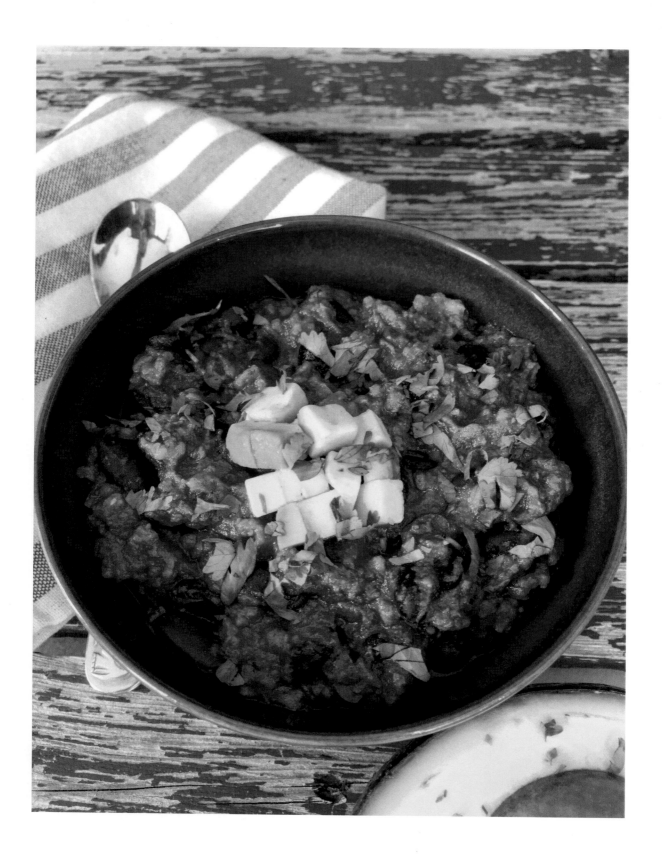

Cool Beans Chili

When heading into a busy go-go weekend with sports, activities, and other events, we love to make this recipe mid-week because it always tastes better the next day. Leftovers can easily be reinvented into tacos or chili "cheese" nachos. Adding avocado and different types of salsa allows for different flavour profiles in the following days.

Gluten-free   Ready in 60 minutes   Makes 12 cups

1 (19 oz) can black beans or 1 cup dry black beans, cook, strain, and rinse (see chart on page xix)

1 (19 oz) can kidney beans or 1 cup dry kidney beans, cook, strain, and rinse (see chart on page xix)

3 stalks celery, diced

1 medium onion, diced

2 cloves garlic, minced

1 medium bell pepper, diced

4-5 mushrooms, diced

2 (28 oz) cans diced or whole tomatoes

2 cups fresh spinach

½ cup homemade BBQ sauce (optional, see page 69 for recipe)

⅔ cup long grain brown rice, dry

1 avocado, diced

2 tbsp avocado oil

1 tbsp chili powder

½ tsp cumin

¼ tsp paprika

¼ tsp coriander

cilantro for garnish

sea salt and pepper to taste

In a large pot, heat oil over medium heat. Sauté the onions, mushroom, peppers, celery, and sea salt, and pepper for 6 minutes. Add garlic spices and continue cooking for another 5 minutes, stir often.

Add your tomatoes and spinach. Increase heat until the sauce starts to simmer. Once sauce has come to a simmer reduce to medium heat and cook for another 5 minutes, stirring continuously.

Add BBQ sauce. Purée with a stick blender. I usually purée all vegetables in the sauce; it is a good way to increase your child's vegetable consumption.

Add rice, kidney beans, and black beans. The rice will absorb some of the water and allow chili to thicken. Cover and allow to simmer for 30-40 mins, stirring occasionally and checking seasoning.

Garnish with fresh avocado and cilantro. Eat hearty.

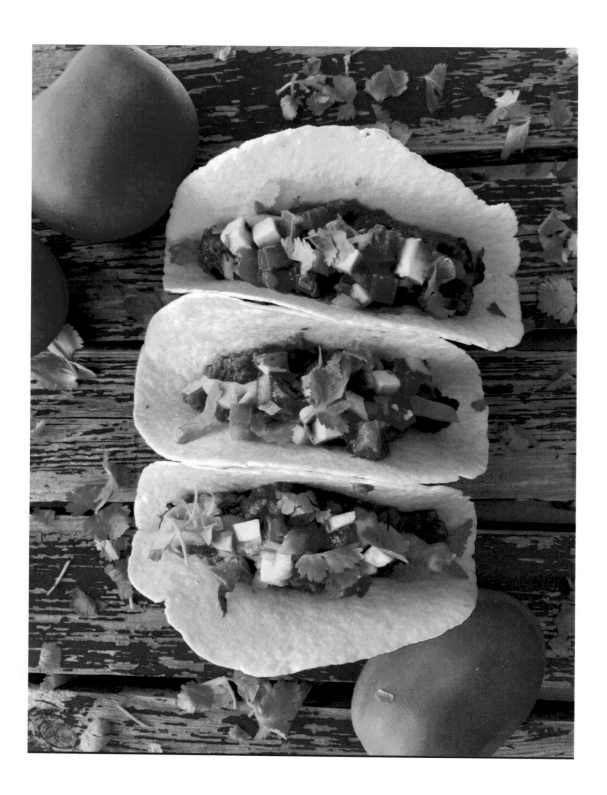

Timeless Tacos

Taco nights are a favourite in our house. We love the versatility and it is a great way to transform leftovers into tasty new meals. Using different types of salsa in place of the tomato and avocado keeps taco nights fun and interesting.

Gluten-free   Ready in 15 minutes   Makes 3 tacos

1 cup Cool Beans Chili (see page 65 for recipe)
3 soft or hard shell tacos, gluten-free
6 tbsp guacamole (see page 51 for recipe)
fresh cilantro for garnish
¼ cup avocado, diced
¼ cup tomato, diced
¼ cup red onion, diced

Roasted Corn Salsa (optional)
1 cup corn kernels, fresh or frozen
¼ cup red pepper, finely diced
¼ cup red onion, finely diced
½ jalapeno, finely diced
1 tsp ginger, grated
1 clove garlic, minced
¼ tsp smoked paprika
juice of ½ lime
1 tbsp avocado oil
1 tbsp cilantro or parsley, chopped

Preheat oven to 350°F.

Begin by preparing or heating up the Cool Beans Chili.

Prepare Guacamole.

Prepare roasted corn salsa, toss corn kernels in oil with pepper and sea salt, and place on baking sheet lined with parchment. Roast for 10 minutes until kernels begin to lightly colour. Remove from heat and cool. Once cooled mix the corn with the remaining ingredients. Makes 12 servings.

Dice avocado, red onion, and tomato. Chop cilantro and set aside.

Warm tacos or wraps in oven.

Place ⅓ cup of chili mixture onto wrap and garnish with 2 tbsp guacamole, 2 tbsp roasted corn salsa (optional), fresh avocado, tomato, red onion, and cilantro. Repeat for additional tacos and serve.

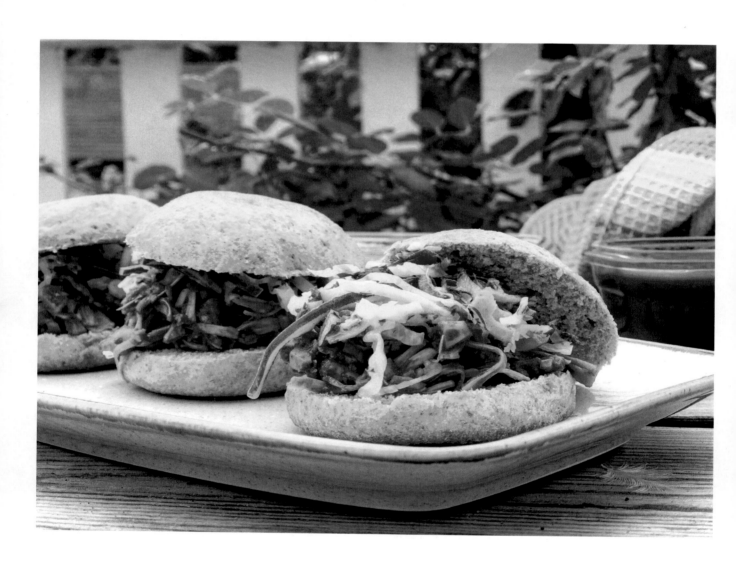

BBQ "You Don't Know" Jackfruit Sliders with Country Slaw

Chad always had a laugh when people compared jackfruit to pulled pork. Being a chef, pulled pork was a dish he had prepared quite often and he just couldn't see the comparison. While on holiday in Hawaii we came across jackfruit and breadfruit almost every day, and soon we tried our first pulled jackfruit sandwich. The resemblance was uncanny. We started out by making this for friends to see if they could tell the difference. We soon perfected a sauce and slaw that brought it all together. This sweet, smoky, and tangy BBQ sauce and crunchy slaw makes the pulled jackfruit a perfect three-bite slider or great on larger kaisers as sandwiches. Blackstrap molasses is high in iron and calcium. Combining it with the Vitamin C found in the tomato sauce increases the absorption of the iron. To make this gluten-free use gluten-free buns.

Ready in 30 minutes   Serves 6

2 (20 oz) cans of young green jackfruit
1 medium onion, diced
1 cup homemade BBQ Sauce
5 tbsp avocado oil
18 slider buns

Country Coleslaw

1 cup green cabbage, shredded
½ cup red cabbage, shredded
¼ cup carrot, peeled and shredded
2 tbsp parsley, chopped
1 tbsp Dijon mustard
1 tbsp agave syrup
1 tbsp lemon juice
1 tbsp rice vinegar
2 tbsp avocado oil
sea salt and pepper to taste

BBQ Sauce

1 (680 ml) can tomato sauce
½ cup apple cider vinegar
¼ cup blackstrap molasses
1 tbsp gluten-free tamari or soy sauce
¼ cup + 2 tbsp demerara sugar,
 firmly packed
5 cloves garlic, minced
1 tbsp smoked sweet paprika
1 ½ tsp ground black pepper
½ tbsp mustard powder
½ tbsp ground coriander
½ tbsp cumin
½ cup apple juice
sea salt to taste
To make this sauce gluten-free use the
 gluten-free tamari

To prepare the BBQ sauce: combine all ingredients. Simmer over medium heat. Take a stick blender and give it a pulse to ensure everything is well-mixed. Whisk continuously to prevent the sauce from burning. Allow to simmer until it is the consistency of BBQ sauce: about 30-35 minutes. Makes 3 cups.

Rinse jackfruit thoroughly; squeeze out excess water. Shred jackfruit in a mini chop or by hand with a knife.

In a large skillet, heat 1 tbsp of oil over medium heat. Add onions and cook over medium heat for about 5 minutes, until onions are translucent. Add another 4 tbsp of oil, jackfruit, sea salt, and pepper to taste. Allow to cook until jackfruit starts to brown. Add BBQ sauce.

While Jackfruit is cooking, prepare your coleslaw. We usually use a mandolin when shaving or shredding the cabbage but using a knife works just as well. Combine the cabbage, carrot, and parsley. In a small bowl, add the Dijon, agave, lemon juice, and rice vinegar. Whisk together, then slowly add your oil while whisking. Once all oil is whisked in, set aside until you are ready to serve the jackfruit before dressing the cabbage. This will prevent the slaw from becoming soggy. When ready, drizzle the dressing over your cabbage and mix well; season with sea salt and cracked pepper. Set aside for topping your jackfruit.

Start building your sandwich: bun, jackfruit, coleslaw and bun. Repeat as needed and enjoy!

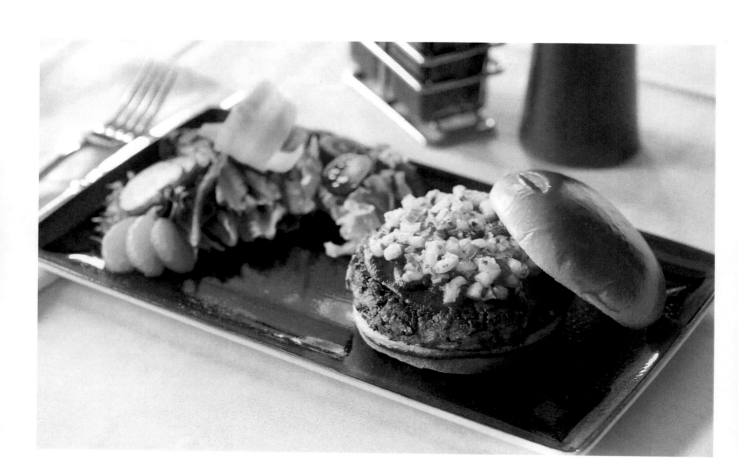

Pacific Coast Black Bean Burgers with Pineapple Salsa

Classic BBQ'd burgers are a must throughout the summer, and we really wanted to create something not only good but fun and different. We noticed how popular vegetable burgers were becoming and how good some places were doing them. This black bean burger holds up well when cooking on the grill or in a pan, and blends the sweet tangy spices of the salsa and BBQ sauce with the rich, earthy beans. We usually have this on the menu twice a week in July and August. Adding smashed avocado or tomato jam is always a nice touch, too. This dish easily becomes gluten-free when you use gluten-free rolled oats and buns.

Ready in 45 minutes   Serves 4

1 (19 oz) can black beans or 1 cup dry black beans, cook, strain, and rinse (see chart on page xix)
½ medium onion, diced
¼ bell pepper, diced
2 cloves garlic, minced
1 tsp cumin
1 tsp coriander
1 tsp paprika
½ cup parsley, chopped
¼ cup rolled oats, gluten-free
¼ cup flax meal
1 tbsp water
sea salt and pepper to taste
¼ cup BBQ sauce
4 burger buns

Pineapple Salsa

½ pineapple, cored, peeled, small diced
½ red pepper, small diced
½ red onion, small diced
3 tbsp fresh cilantro, chopped
2 tbsp extra virgin olive oil
1 tbsp fresh ginger, minced
1 clove garlic, minced
1 jalapeno, small diced
1-2 limes, juiced
sea salt and pepper to taste

Cook the black beans and let cool.

While beans are cooling, prepare the pineapple salsa. In a bowl mix all ingredients gently and season. If you can, prepare the pineapple salsa the night before. Allowing it to marinate overnight will intensify the flavours. Makes 6 servings.

Using a potato masher or fork, mash up the beans.

Add rolled oats, flax meal, water, onions, bell pepper, garlic, parsley, spices, sea salt, and pepper. Mix together using hands.

Set the black bean burgers aside in fridge and let chill for 30 minutes. This will help the burger patties firm up and hold together better.

On medium heat, preheat frying pan with oil. Fry burgers for 5-6 minutes per side.

Once cooked build your burger: bun, burger, 1 tbsp BBQ sauce, pineapple salsa, and bun. Repeat as needed.

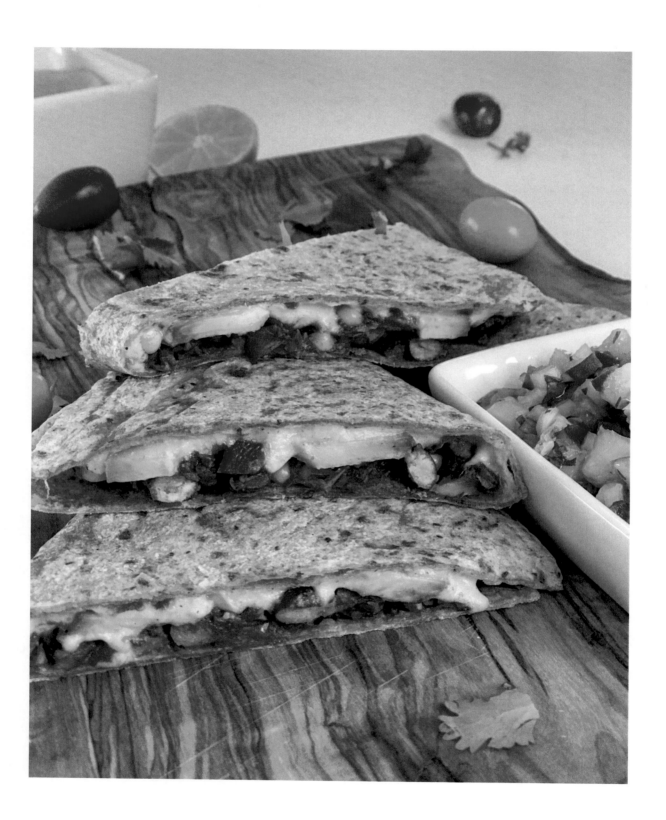

Bean & Avocado Cashewdillas with Peach Salsa

This is a classic pub snack: crunchy, crispy, melted, and stretchy cheese. The vegan cheese bears such a resemblance in taste and texture it really makes this a favourite even with our non-vegan friends. To make this gluten-free use gluten-free tortilla wraps.

Ready in 45 minutes   Serves 4

1 (15 oz) can kidney beans or ¾ cup dry kidney beans, cook, strain, and rinse (see chart on page xix)
⅔ cup onions, diced
¾ cup bell pepper, diced
1 cup mushrooms, sliced
1 ear of corn
½ cup vegetable stock
1 tbsp avocado oil
1 cup tomato, diced
½ lime, juiced
1 avocado, sliced
1 tsp chili powder
½ tsp smoked paprika
1 clove garlic, minced
¼ tsp onion powder
½ tsp cumin
¼ tsp crushed chilies
cilantro to garnish
sea salt and pepper to taste
4 tortilla wraps

Peach Salsa

2 peaches, diced small
3 tbsp cilantro, chopped
¼ red onion, diced small
1 tbsp fresh ginger, minced
½ jalapeno, diced small
½ lime, juiced
½ red pepper, diced small
dash of sea salt

Vegan Cheese

1/2 cup raw cashews
1/4 cup tapioca flour/starch
1 tsp lime juice
1 ¼ cup vegetable stock or water
1 ½ tbsp nutritional yeast
½ tsp sea salt
½ tsp garlic powder
½ tsp onion powder
¼ tsp chili powder
¼ tsp pepper

Soak cashews for 3 hours or overnight. If you haven't prepped ahead, pour boiling water over them and let sit for 15-20 minutes.

Strain the cashews. In a blender, add the cashews, vegetable stock, tapioca flour, lime juice, nutritional yeast, sea salt, pepper, and spices. Purée ingredients on high speed for 2 minutes.

Pour the cashew mixture in a small saucepan over medium heat. Cook for 3-5 minutes until the cheese forms into a gooey ball in the centre. Stir constantly to prevent sticking. The cheese will stay fairly soft and sticky. Remove from heat and set aside.

In a large skillet heat oil over medium heat. Sauté the onions, mushroom, corn, and peppers; season with sea salt and pepper. After 3 minutes add garlic and spices. Continue cooking for another 3-4 minutes until onions are translucent. Stir often to prevent from sticking. Add vegetable stock, lime juice, and kidney beans. Let it simmer and reduce.

While filling is cooking, prepare peach salsa. Combine all ingredients and mix gently.

Once vegetable stock has reduced, add tomatoes and cook for another couple of minutes. Tip: If the liquid hasn't reduced, the filling will be too wet and make the quesadillas soggy. Once it's done, turn the heat off and fill the quesadillas.

Spread vegan cheese on one half and spread the bean filling on the other. Garnish with cilantro and sliced avocado. Fold tortilla in half. In a non-stick frying pan over medium heat, cook the quesadilla for approximately 45 seconds on each side until the tortillas are crispy and the cheese is melted. Cut into triangles and serve with peach salsa.

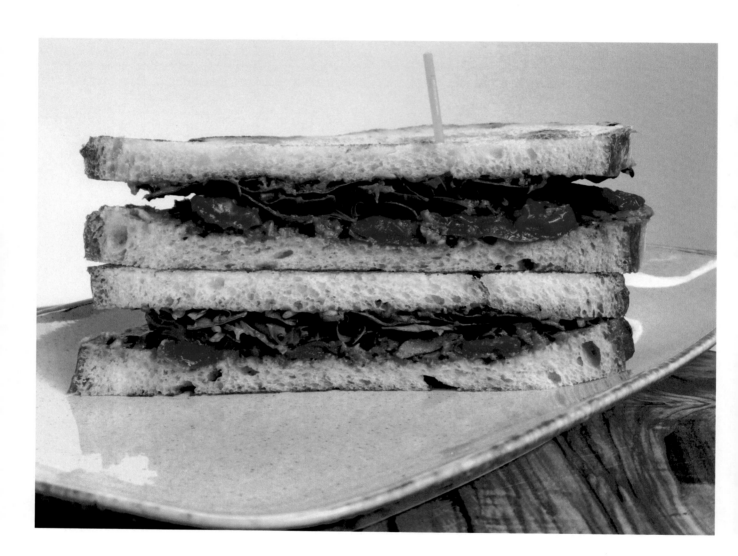

Oven Roasted Eggplant & Tomato Panini

I love having a panini or baba ganoush for lunch or a snack and this recipe brings them both together. We've added the sweet and smoky roasted tomatoes, which goes well with the spice of arugula, on this sandwich and we always seem to have an eggplant on hand for a lazy weekend lunch.

Ready in 55 minutes   Serves 4

2 cups grape tomatoes
2 cups arugula
1 loaf French bread, sliced
1 ½ tbsp extra virgin olive oil
1-2 tsp vegan butter
sea salt and pepper to taste

Eggplant Spread

1 large eggplant
4 cloves garlic, roasted
½ cup parsley
1 ½ tbsp extra virgin olive oil
½ lemon juice
2 tbsp nutritional yeast

Preheat oven to 325°F. Line baking sheet with parachment paper.

Slice the eggplant and tomatoes in half lengthwise. Place both on a baking sheet skins down and drizzle with olive oil, sea salt, and pepper. Add garlic (skins on) to the baking sheet and roast.

Remove garlic from the oven after about 18-20 minutes. Continue roasting the tomatoes and eggplant for 15-20 minutes.

For the roasted eggplant spread, combine eggplant, peeled garlic, parsley, lemon, and nutritional yeast in a bowl and purée with a stick blender or food processor.

Take 2 slices of French bread, and butter one side of each with a vegan butter. On the other side, spread eggplant spread, then place tomatoes and arugula. Heat a frying pan on medium heat and grill your sandwich until brown. Remove from heat, cut, and serve.

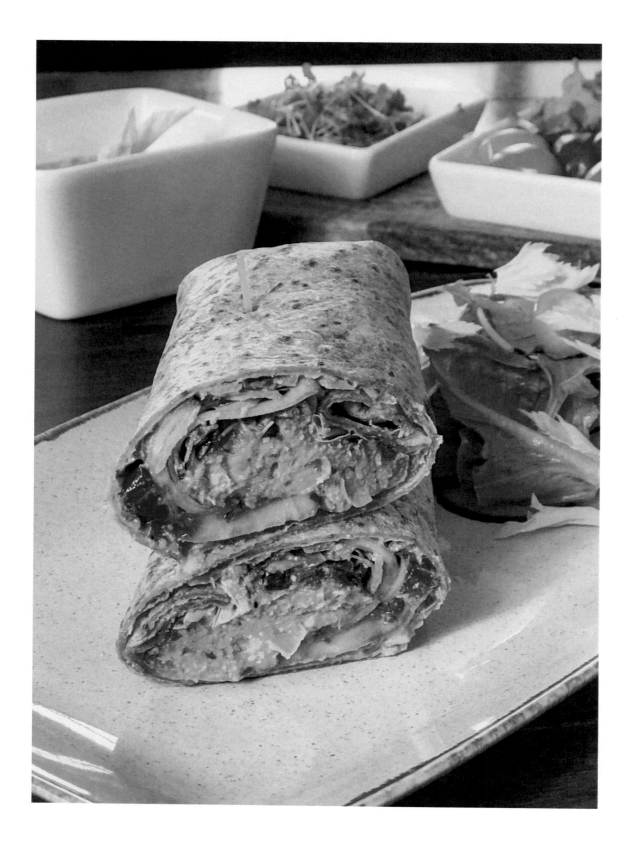

Tahini & Lentil Falafel Wrap with Roasted Red Pepper Dressing

This recipe was inspired by a dish we had while on holiday in London, England. Serving this with a side of the red pepper dressing or a coconut yogurt tzatziki for dipping makes a perfect accompaniment. This dish can easily be gluten-free by using gluten-free wraps or by making a deconstructed wrap. To make a deconstructed wrap add greens, cucumber, grape tomatoes, grilled zucchini, red onions, and falafels in a bowl; finish by topping it with the roasted red pepper dressing.

Ready in 45-55 minutes   Serves 5

Falafel

1 heaping cup can chickpeas or ½ cup dry chickpeas, cook, strain, and rinse (see chart on page xix)
1 cup red lentils, dry
1 tsp cumin
1 tsp coriander
1 tsp turmeric
1 tsp smoked paprika
3 cloves garlic, minced
1 tbsp extra virgin olive oil
1 small onion, finely diced
2 tbsp water added to spice and onions while frying
⅔ cup fresh parsley or dill
2 tbsp lemon juice
1 tsp lemon zest
2 tbsp tahini
2 tbsp hemp seeds
sea salt and pepper to taste
2 ½ cups arugula
broccoli sprouts for garnish (optional)
2 carrots, peeled and grated
1 tomato, sliced
½ cumber, sliced
5 wraps

Roasted Red Pepper Dressing

2 roasted red peppers
2 cloves roasted garlic
¼ tsp onion powder
2 tbsp lemon juice
¼ cup cashews (soak overnight or soak in boiling water for 15- 20 minutes)
sea salt and pepper to taste

Preheat oven to 400°F. Line a baking sheet with parchment paper.

Cut red peppers in half and place them skin up on a baking sheet. Place garlic on the baking sheet and place in the oven.

After approximately 5 minutes, remove garlic from the oven. Roast red peppers for about 20-25 minutes. You want the skin to become wrinkled and blackened. Once they are done, pull them out, set aside, and let cool.

While red peppers are in the oven, cook red lentils (see chart on page xix). Strain and set aside to cool.

In a small frying pan, heat oil over medium heat. Add onions and sauté for 6-8 minutes until onions become translucent.

Add cumin, coriander, turmeric, smoked paprika, and garlic, and sauté for 1 minute. Add water to create a paste. Then remove from heat. If you want to save time you can add the onion and spices raw, but we find sautéing the onions and spices enhances the flavours.

Using a stick blender or food processor, break down the chickpeas and red lentils by pulsing. Add onion and the spice mixture, tahini, lemon juice, hemp seeds, and fresh parsley. Season with sea salt and pepper.

Adjust oven to 350°F. Line baking sheet with parchment paper; mould falafel mixture into 2-inch round cakes. Bake in oven for 10-12 minutes. Makes 15 falafels.

While falafels are in the oven, prepare roasted red pepper dressing. Peel roasted red peppers and garlic. Rinse and drain cashews. Add roasted red pepper, garlic, cashews, lemon juice, onion powder, sea salt, and pepper to the blender and purée. One serving equals ¼ cup.

Warm your wraps or tortillas in the oven. Once removed, begin building the wraps. Add red pepper dressing, arugula, sliced tomato, cucumber, and broccoli sprouts, and top with 3 falafel cakes. Drizzle with a little more dressing. Wrap them up folding in the ends as you go, slice in half, and enjoy.

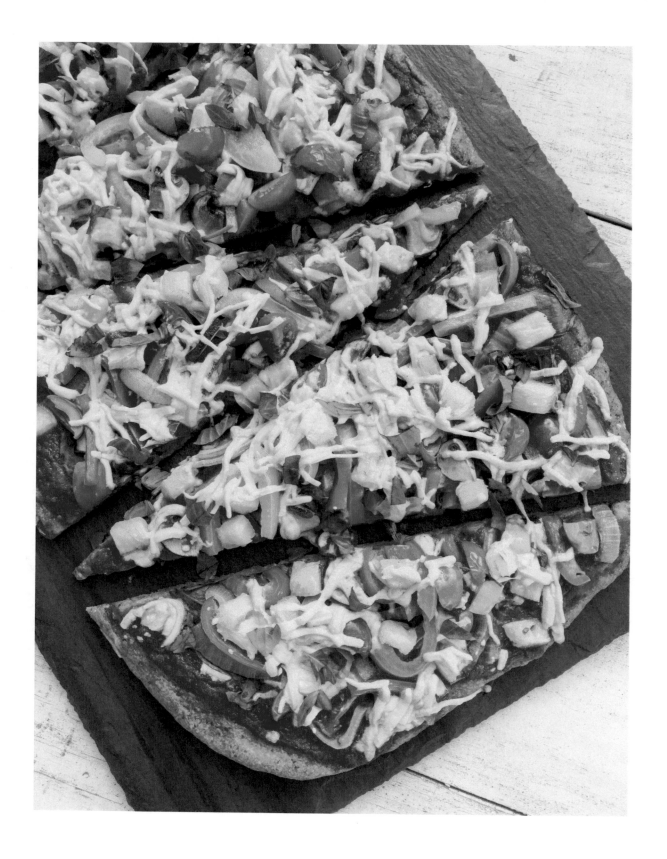

Sprouted Spelt Flour Pizza

Who doesn't love pizza night? Especially, when it is homemade. Changing up toppings and making your own personal pizza allows for all to play a role in the outcome of dinner. River gets his classic green olive and pineapple and then we can switch ours up each time. Smoked tempeh is a great bacon alternative.

Using an ancient grain—spelt flour—is lower in gluten and higher in protein. It gives the dough a crispy, lighter crust compared to a whole wheat flour. Being sprouted also makes it easier on the digestive system.

The secret to a crispy dough is high heat for a shorter amount of time. Also, we usually make this without the non-dairy cheese and it tastes great. Cheese is completely optional.

Ready in 1 hour 10 minutes   Makes 12 slices

½ cup red pepper, julienned
½ cup yellow pepper, julienned
1 cup red onion, julienned
1 ¼ cup mushrooms, diced
⅓ cup green olives, diced into quarters
1 cup grape tomatoes, diced into quarters
1 cup pineapple, finely diced
2 cups marinara sauce (see page 81
    for recipe)
3 cups spinach
1 package of non-dairy mozzarella (optional)
fresh basil to garnish

Sprouted Spelt Flour Dough

2 ¾ cups sprouted or regular spelt flour
¼ cup flax meal
1 ⅓ cup of warm water
1 tbsp turbinado sugar
2 ¼ tsp yeast
1 tsp of sea salt
¼ cup olive oil

Prepare dough. Mix together water, sugar, and yeast until mixture turns cloudy then let sit for 10 minutes until a good foam has formed on top. In a large bowl, mix spelt flour, flax meal, and sea salt. Pour in the water and yeast mixture. Knead and add olive oil. Knead until everything is mixed smooth then cover the bowl with plastic wrap and let rise for 45 minutes-1 hour.

While dough is rising, prepare your vegetables.

Preheat oven to 400°F. Cut dough into 2 equal balls. Lay down parchment paper on a baking sheet. Place your dough in the middle of the paper and roll out. If the dough is sticking to your hands, dust dough lightly with flour.

Spread marinara over the dough, lay down spinach and the rest of the vegetables, and cover with non-dairy cheese.

Place in oven and bake for 5 minutes. Remove pizza from baking sheet and lay it (with parchment paper) directly on the oven rack. Bake for an additional 5-8 minutes. One serving equals one slice.

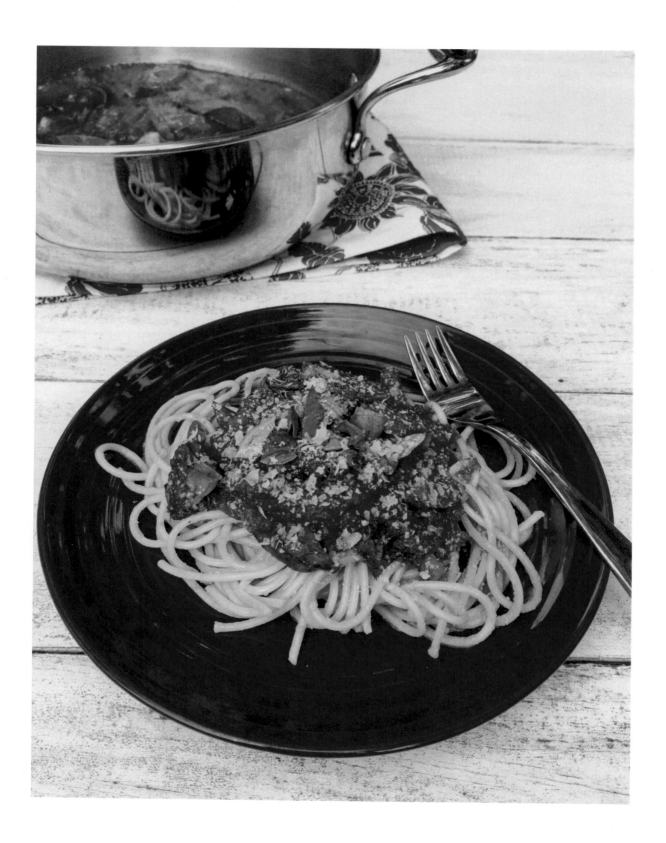

Pronto Pasta Primavera

This is a recipe I always make more than needed because it can be used for so many other recipes and meals. A pasta night followed by a pizza night makes for an easy few days of meal planning. Adding nutritional yeast adds a nice nutty flavour that mimics parmesan cheese and is often fortified with B vitamins. For a gluten-free meal use gluten-free pasta.

Ready in 30 minutes   Serves 6

1 red pepper, diced
1 small red onion, diced
½ zucchini, diced
4 mushrooms, diced
2 cups spinach
1 tbsp extra virgin olive oil
3 cups marinara sauce (see recipe below)
fresh basil
12 tsp nutritional yeast
450 g pasta

Marinara Sauce
2 cloves garlic, minced
2 (28 oz) can tomatoes
1 (6 oz) can tomato paste
1 tbsp extra virgin olive oil
3 stalks celery, diced
1 medium onion, diced
3 tsp Italian seasoning
2 bay leaves
sea salt and pepper to taste

To prepare the marinara sauce, heat a large pot with oil over medium heat. Sauté onions, celery, sea salt, and pepper for 5 minutes. Add garlic and continue to sauté for another minute.

Add tomatoes, tomato paste, and Italian seasoning. Bring to a simmer and purée with stick blender. Add bay leaf and simmer for 15-20 minutes. Makes 7 cups.

Bring a large pot of salted water to a boil. Cook pasta as per instructions on the package. Strain and set aside.

In a large saucepan, heat oil over medium heat. Add red pepper, red onion, zucchini, mushroom, sea salt, and pepper to taste. Sauté for approximately 7 minutes until onions are translucent.

Add 3 cups of marinara and let simmer for a few minutes. Stir in spinach; cook until spinach is wilted. Check seasoning.

Serve pasta topped with sauce. Sprinkle with 2 tsp nutritional yeast and fresh basil (optional).

Once marinara has cooled, store in the fridge for the homemade pizza or freeze.

Tip
When cooking pasta always salt the water; it will bring out the flavour. Many people add oil to the water when cooking pasta, but if you have the time there is no need to; some say it does more harm than good. Gently stir your pasta as it is added to the boiling water, and every so often repeat; this will help break up the starches in the pasta and prevent the noodles from clinging to each other.

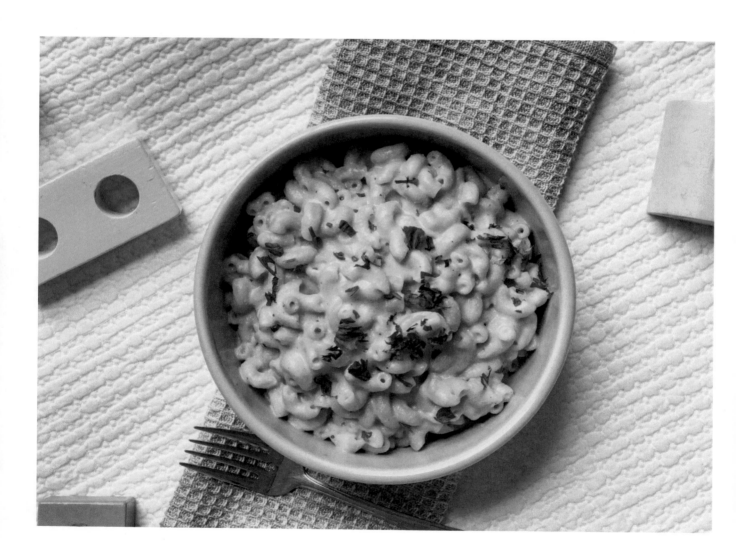

Return of the Mac 'n' Cheese

We both wanted to replicate this classic kid favourite but wondered how we could replicate a cheesy taste and texture. We tried many ways with a roux and with other cheese substitutes but nothing came close. In this recipe, the coconut and cashews add a nuttiness comparable with certain cheeses. The nutritional yeast and potato also add a parmesan taste and texture. For a gluten-free meal use gluten-free macaroni.

Ready in 25 minutes   Serves 4

2 ½ cups macaroni, dry
½ cup onion, finely diced
1 tbsp garlic, minced
1 tbsp vegan butter or oil
1 cup potato, peeled and small diced
½ cup cashews
1 cup unsweetened almond milk
½ cup canned coconut milk
¼ cup vegetable stock or water
⅛ tsp nutmeg
¼ tsp onion powder
¼ tsp garlic powder
⅛ tsp smoked paprika
3 tbsp nutritional yeast
sea salt and pepper to taste
fresh parsley or broccoli florets to garnish (optional)

Bring a medium pot of salted water to boil, add macaroni, and cook as per directions on box. Strain and add a splash of oil and combine. This will prevent the macaroni from sticking together. Set aside.

Heat a small sauce pot with oil or vegan butter over medium heat. Add onions and sauté until they begin to brown and caramelize. Add the minced garlic, cook for 2 minutes, and add all the dry spices except the nutritional yeast. Mix well and add the vegetable stock followed by almond milk, coconut milk, potatoes, and cashews. Gently simmer over low heat until potatoes are cooked and cashews have softened. Remove from heat.

Cool mixture for a few minutes before puréeing. Once mixture has cooled down a little, pour it into blender and purée. Add nutritional yeast and blend once more.

Pour sauce back into the sauce pot and add your cooked macaroni. Mix well and garnish with parsley or roasted broccoli florets and dig in.

Tip
When cooking pasta always salt the water; it will bring out the flavour. Many people add oil to the water when cooking pasta, but if you have the time there is no need to; some say it does more harm than good. Gently stir your pasta as it is added to the boiling water, and every so often repeat; this will help break up the starches in the pasta and prevent the noodles from clinging to each other.

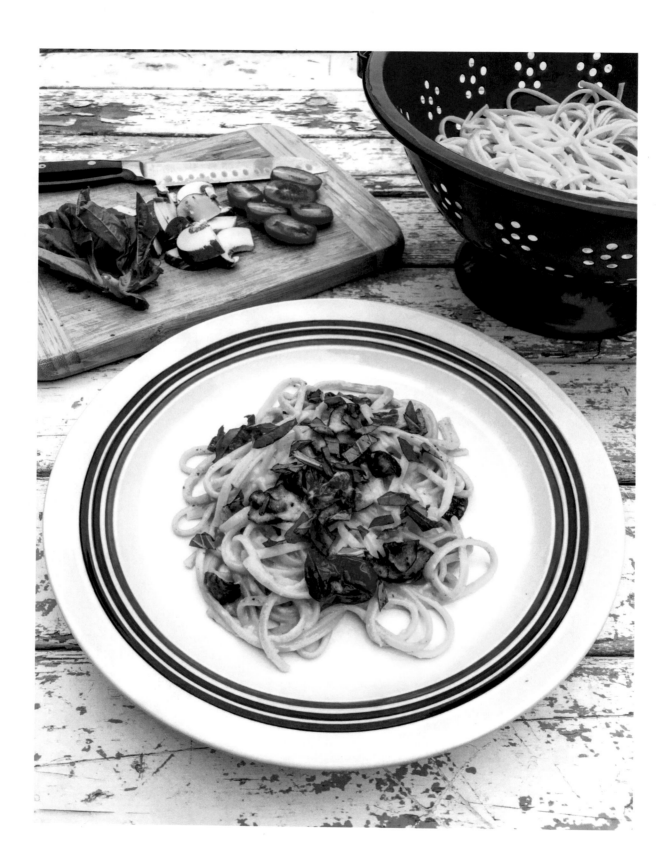

Oven Roasted Tomato & Mushroom Alfredo

When we first transitioned to a plant-based diet, pasta became a common dish. We eventually realized we missed the flavours of a rich, creamy Alfredo sauce, but we did not miss the feeling of being weighed down and bloated after consuming it. This is similar to the mac 'n' cheese recipe, except we deglaze with a local white wine and add roasted garlic to this sauce. In the fall, we substitute the potato for parsnips or squash, filling the house with sweet fall aromas. For a gluten-free option use gluten-free pasta.

Ready in 45-55 minutes   Serves 6

20 grape tomatoes
3 cups mushrooms, sliced
1 medium onion, diced
5 cloves garlic
1 cup cooked potato
1 cup cooked parsnip
4 tbsp extra virgin olive oil
⅓ cup raw cashews
½ cup white wine
1 ½ cups unsweetened almond milk
1 ½ cups vegetable stock
2 tbsp nutritional yeast
fresh basil
450 g of pasta
sea salt and pepper to taste

Preheat oven to 325°F. Line a baking sheet with parchment paper.

Slice tomatoes lengthwise and lay them with the sliced side face up on a baking sheet. Drizzle approximately 1 tbsp of extra virgin olive oil over the tomatoes and season with salt and pepper.

In a medium mixing bowl, add the sliced mushrooms, toss in 2 tbsp of extra virgin olive oil, and season with sea salt and pepper to taste. Add to baking sheet along with the garlic (peels on) and place in the oven.

Peel and dice 1 cup potato and 1 cup parsnip.

After 18-20 minutes, remove the garlic and mushrooms from the baking sheet, place the tomatoes back in the oven, and roast for another 15-20 minutes.

To prepare the Alfredo sauce: In a medium saucepan, heat 1 tbsp of extra virgin olive oil over medium heat. Add onions and sauté for a few minutes, seasoning with sea salt and pepper to taste. Deglaze the onions with white wine and reduce with a gentle simmer. Peel the roasted garlic and add it to the onions and wine; simmer for 3 minutes. Once the white wine has reduced, add the vegetable stock, cashews, potato, and parsnip; bring to a boil and reduce to simmer. Add almond milk and continue simmering for 18-20 minutes until potato and parsnip have softened enough to purée. Remove from heat and add nutritional yeast, sea salt, and pepper.

Purée using a blender or stick blender. If needed you can add more vegetable stock or almond milk to adjust thickness to desired consistency.

Bring a large pot of salted water to a boil and cook pasta as directed on package. Strain and set aside in a large pot.

Add the mushrooms and tomatoes to the Alfredo sauce and stir in. Pour sauce over pasta and garnish with torn garden basil.

Tip

When cooking pasta always salt the water; it will bring out the flavour. Many people add oil to the water when cooking pasta, but if you have the time there is no need to; some say it does more harm than good. Gently stir your pasta as it is added to the boiling water, and every so often repeat; this will help break up the starches in the pasta and prevent the noodles from clinging to each other.

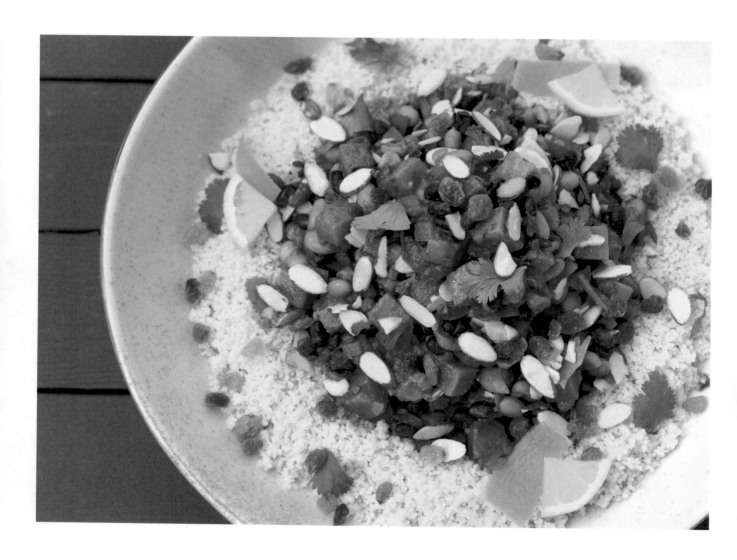

Moroccan Sweet Potato & Black Bean Tagine

Travel is what we look forward to the most in our family. We love spending time together checking out new destinations whether it's a day road trip, longer stays overnight, or trips to other countries. The most exciting element is checking out the local food scene or craft and farmer's markets. It is important to appreciate where ingredients come from and how they are prepared in different cultures. Our plant-based tagine begins with our play on the famous "Ras el hanout" Moroccan spice mixture (which means "top shelf" or "top shop"), minus the heat of the cayenne pepper and the herb fenugreek. We've added sweet potato, black beans, crisp chickpeas, and almonds for texture, and we serve it on top of warm couscous, topped with fresh cilantro and plump golden raisins. We love to break this recipe out when entertaining friends or family, and then we take everyone on a trip around our dining table.

To keep this recipe gluten-free, use rice or quinoa in place of the couscous. Using dried apricots, cherries, or cranberries also works well in place of the raisins.

Ready in 1 hour   Serves 6

1 (19 oz) can black beans, drained or 1 cup dry black beans, cook, strain, and rinse (see chart on page xix)
1 (19 oz) can white beans, drained, or 1 cup dry white beans, cook, strain, and rinse (see chart on page xix)
1 (19 oz) can chickpeas, drained, or 1 cup dry chickpeas, cook, strain, and rinse (see chart on page xix)
1 medium onion, diced
1 cup celery, diced
4-5 cloves garlic, minced
2 cups sweet potato, peeled and diced
1 tbsp fresh ginger, minced
2 vine tomatoes, diced
1 cup golden raisins (½ cup for garnish, ½ cup in the tagine)
1 tbsp sliced almonds
1 tbsp parsley, chopped
2 tbsp cilantro, chopped (reserve 1 tbsp for garnish)
5 tbsp Moroccan spice (see recipe below)
4 cups vegetable stock
1 tbsp + 1 tsp of extra virgin olive oil
1 cup couscous, dry
½ lemon for garnish
sea salt and pepper to taste

Moroccan Spice

1 tbsp allspice
1 tbsp cinnamon
2 tbsp cumin
2 tbsp garlic powder
1 tbsp onion powder
2 tbsp ginger powder
2 tsp coriander
1 tbsp smoked paprika
1 tbsp turmeric
½ tbsp ground clove
1 tbsp cardamom
1 tbsp sea salt
1 tbsp black pepper

Preheat oven to 400°F. Line a baking sheet with parchment paper.

In a small frying pan over medium heat, toast Moroccan spice mixture for 3 minutes, gently tossing to help release flavours and aromas. Cool spice mixture and place in Ziploc bag or airtight container for future use.

Place chickpeas in a small bowl with 1 tsp of olive oil and 3 tsp of Moroccan spice mixture. Toss until evenly coated.

Spread evenly over baking sheet and roast for 15 minutes. Roll chickpeas around and place back in oven for another 15-20 minutes, until they are dehydrated and crunchy. Cool and reserve half for garnish and the other for a snack.

For the Moroccan Bean and Sweet Potato Tagine:

Warm a large pot with 1 tbsp oil over medium heat and sauté your onions and celery for 2-3 minutes. Add tomato, garlic, and ginger; continue sautéing until the onions begin to soften and brown, about 3-5 minutes. Add 2 tbsp of the Moroccan spice mix and stir in well.

Add vegetable stock, bring to boil, and reduce to simmer. Add sweet potato and 3 more tbsp of Moroccan spice mixture, parsley, and cilantro. Allow to simmer for 15-20 minutes or until the sweet potato becomes soft and the flavours have all come together.

Add cooked black beans, white beans, and raisins. Mix well. Check seasoning.

Remove from heat. We garnish with sliced and blanched almonds, golden raisins, roasted chickpeas, chopped cilantro, and ½ of a fresh lemon juiced and zested over top. We serve with the couscous on the bottom and the tagine on top, followed by the garnish.

For the couscous, place 1 cup of couscous in a stainless-steel bowl or pan, and pour 1 ½ cups of boiling water or vegetable stock over it. Cover with plastic wrap and let steep for 8-10 minutes. Once couscous has steeped, remove the wrap and gently run a fork through it. This will help separate the couscous and fluff up the grains.

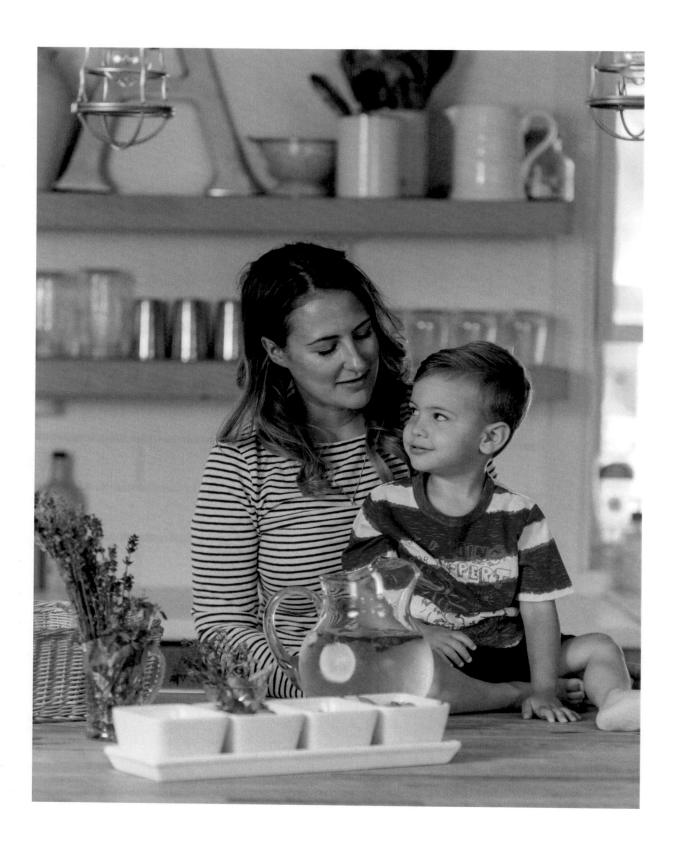

SWEET STREET

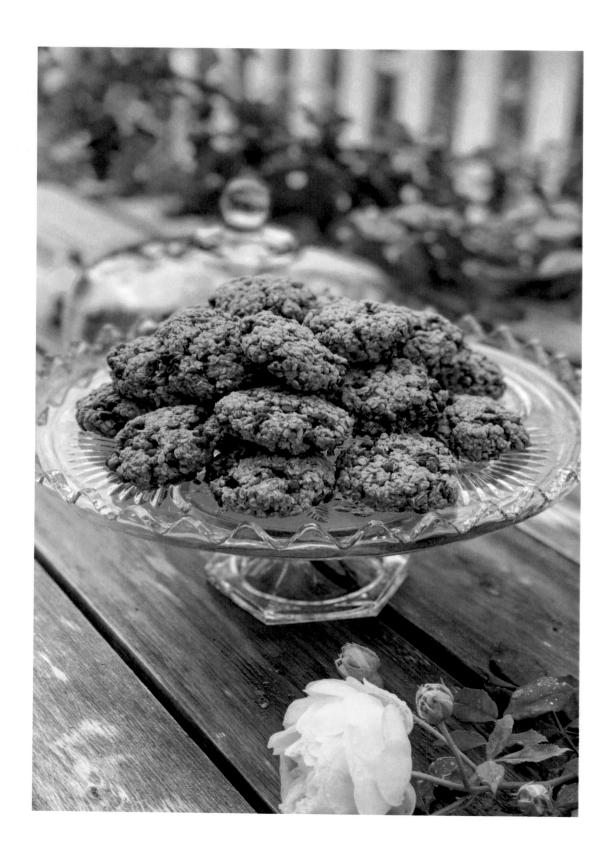

Nanny's Oatmeal Chocolate Chip Cookies

Some of our earliest cooking memories are baking with our grandmothers. To this day, baking is one of my favourite pastimes. One of the reasons I love to bake is I can make healthier treats for the family. A couple of ways I achieve this is by using natural sweetener or sugar that has been minimally refined, and whole grain/sprouted spelt flour in place of all-purpose flour. These are one of my grandmother's amazing recipes that I have tweaked by eliminating animal products and reducing the amount of sugar. These cookies are super quick and easy to make. You wouldn't even know that this recipe has been altered; it's just as good as Nanny's.

Ready in 30 minutes   Makes 24 cookies

¾ cup vegan butter, softened
¾ cup demerara sugar
¼ cup turbinado sugar
1 tbsp flax meal + 3 tbsp water
2 tbsp water
2 tsp pure vanilla extract
1 tsp cinnamon
¾ tsp baking soda
3 cups quick rolled oats
¾ cup spelt flour
1 cup vegan chocolate chips

Preheat oven to 350°F. Line a baking tray with parchment paper.

Prepare egg replacer. Mix 1 tbsp flax meal in 3 tbsp water. Let sit for 5 minutes until it has thickened.

In a medium bowl, cream together sugars, butter, and egg replacer. Add remaining wet ingredients.

In a large bowl, combine dry ingredients and mix well. Pour wet mixture in with dry ingredients and stir together.

Fold in chocolate chips. Mould dough into round little balls and place on the baking tray.

Bake for 15 minutes. Remove from oven and place on cooling rack.

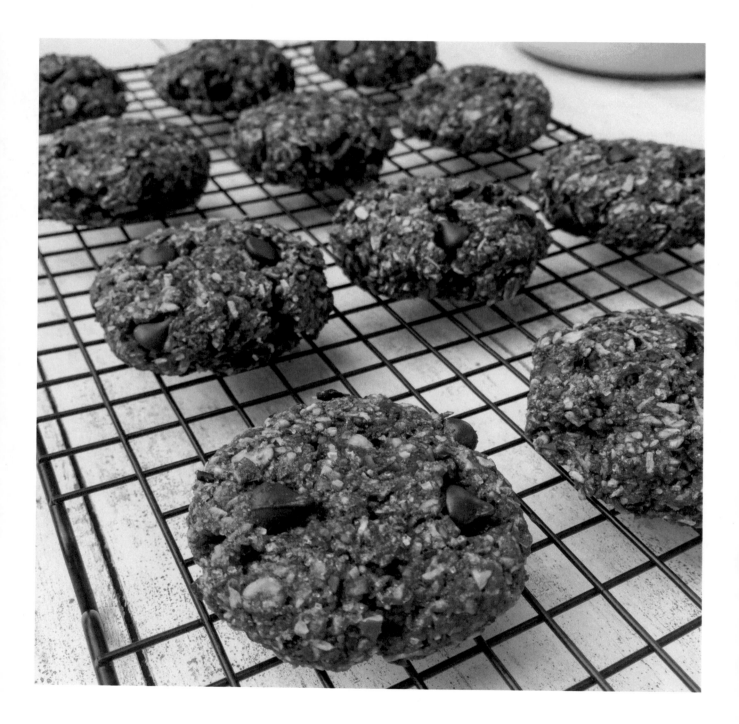

High Vibing Bean & Molasses Cookies

The cookie that eats like a meal. I know it sounds funny, but seriously, these cookies are loaded with nuts, seeds, and beans, which makes them high in fibre. We've added blackstrap molasses, which helps with the flavour but it is also high in iron and calcium. Usually something that sounds like this is too good to be true. Not the case here. These are some of the best cookies we've ever made, taste and health-wise, by far. It's the kind of cookie that leaves no guilt if ever needed for a bribe, not that we've ever done that.

Ready in 35 minutes   Makes 15 cookies

¾ cup rolled oats
½ cup shredded unsweetened coconut
½ cup spelt flour
¼ cup pumpkin seeds
⅓ cup sunflower seeds
1 heaping cup can black beans, drained or ½ cup dry black beans, cook, strain, and rinse (see chart on page xix)
1 tsp cinnamon
¼ tsp nutmeg
2 tbsp blackstrap molasses
¼ cup coconut oil
1 tbsp flax meal + 3 tbsp water
½ cup coconut sugar
½ tsp baking soda
⅓ cup chocolate chips
pinch of sea salt

Preheat oven to 350°F. Line a baking tray with parchment paper.

Prepare egg replacer. Mix 1 tbsp of flax meal in 3 tbsp of water. Let sit for 5 minutes until it has thickened.

In a blender, pulse pumpkin seeds, sunflower seeds, and rolled oats until they are coarsely ground (if you use quick oats you don't need to grind them. If you pulse the seed into a fine ground you will have to add 2 tbsp of water to the dough).

In a large bowl, sift together spelt flour and baking soda (to remove lumps). Combine seeds, oats, cinnamon, nutmeg, coconut, and sea salt. Stir.

In a medium mixing bowl, mix sugar, molasses, egg replacer, and melted coconut oil.

In a separate bowl use a stick blender and purée black beans. Combine black beans to the wet ingredients and mix well.

Pour wet mixture in the large bowl with the dry ingredients and stir together. Fold in chocolate chips.

Mould cookie dough into balls on the baking sheet. Bake for 14-15 minutes. Remove from oven and place on a cooling rack.

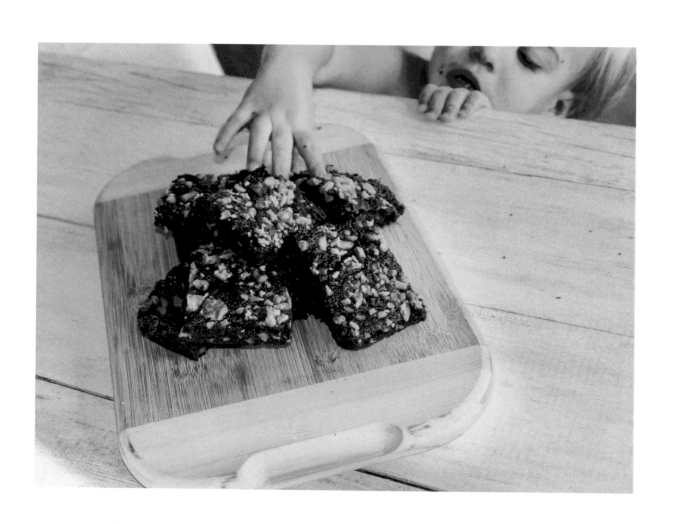

"No Frownies with these Brownies"

Caught with their hands in the brownie jar! Once these delicious treats are made—even if still warm or packed away nicely—hands will be caught in the brownie jar. It's hard to keep these treats around, so if I'm ever making these for special events or parties I usually end up having to hide these tasty bites before they disappear. They are dense and soft but with crunchy walnuts evenly placed on top, you will soon understand the disappearing brownie epidemic.

Gluten-free   Ready in 40 minutes   Makes 16 squares

1 cup almond flour
¼ cup tapioca flour or starch
¾ cup turbinado sugar
⅓ cup cocoa powder
½ cup coconut oil
½ tsp baking soda
½ cup walnuts, chopped
1 medium banana
1 tbsp flax meal + 2 tbsp water
1 tsp vanilla
pinch of sea salt

Preheat oven to 350°F. Line an 8 x 8 baking dish with parchment paper.

Prepare egg replacer. Mix 1 tbsp of flax meal in 2 tbsp of water. Let sit for 5 minutes until it has thickened.

In a large mixing bowl, sift almond flour, tapioca flour, cocoa powder, and baking soda (to remove lumps). Add salt and mix dry ingredients together.

In a medium mixing bowl, purée banana with a sick blender. Add sugar, coconut oil, egg replacer, and vanilla; mix together with a wooden spoon.

Pour wet ingredients into the large mixing bowl with the dry and stir together.

Pour batter into baking dish and sprinkle the top with walnuts. Bake for 30 minutes. Remove from oven and let cool. Cut and serve.

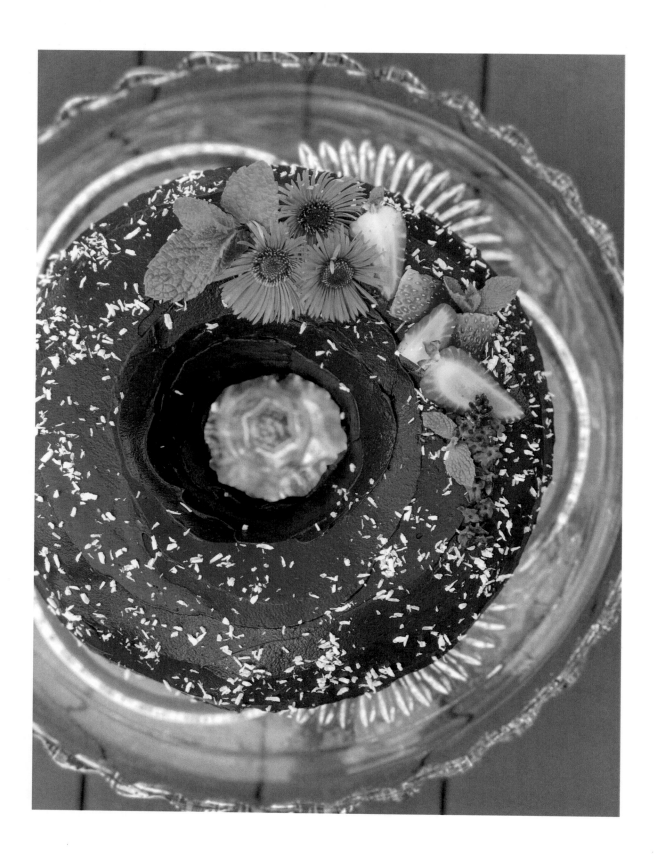

Double Chocolate Cake with Chocolate Avocado Icing

This chocolate cake was my all-time favourite as a kid and still is to this day. We like to call it the "Grandmother of all Cakes" as we've adapted my grandmother's family recipe into a vegan hybrid that uses spelt flour, half the sugar, and an epic avocado icing in place of the traditional buttercream icing. The cake stays super moist and the sweet avocado icing only adds to the rich beauty.

Ready in 1 hour   Serves 12

2 cups spelt flour
1 cup turbinado sugar
1 cup non-dairy milk + 1 tbsp vinegar (buttermilk replacer)
½ cup cocoa
⅔ cup coconut oil
¾ tbsp baking soda
1 tbsp flax meal mixed + 3 tbsp
1 cup hot coffee
¼ cup of shredded coconut for garnish (optional)
pinch of sea salt

Chocolate Avocado Icing
⅓ cup + 2 tbsp icing sugar
⅓ cup cocoa
2 avocados
3 tsp vanilla extract

Preheat oven to 350°F. Grease a Bundt pan.

Prepare egg replacer. Mix 1 tbsp of flax meal in 3 tbsp of water. Let sit for 5 minutes until it has thickened.

Prepare buttermilk replacer by mixing 1 tbsp of vinegar in 1 cup of non-dairy milk.

In a medium bowl, cream together melted coconut oil and sugar. Add buttermilk replacer, egg replacer, and hot coffee. Mix together.

Sift spelt flour, cocoa powder, and baking soda (to remove clumps) into a large mixing bowl. Add sea salt and mix together all the dry ingredients.

Pour the wet ingredients in the large mixing bowl with the dry ingredients. Use an electric mixer or hand beater on medium speed and mix cake batter until smooth. Pour cake batter into the Bundt pan and place into the oven.

Bake for 40-45 minutes. Once cake is baked remove from oven and place on a rack to cool.

While cake is baking, prepare the icing. In a medium bowl, use a stick blender to purée avocados and vanilla extract. Sift in icing sugar and cocoa powder purée.

Once cake has cooled, remove from Bundt pan and ice it. Adding coconut to garnish is optional. We try for 12 servings, but sometimes it turns into 8. Store in a airtight container in the fridge.

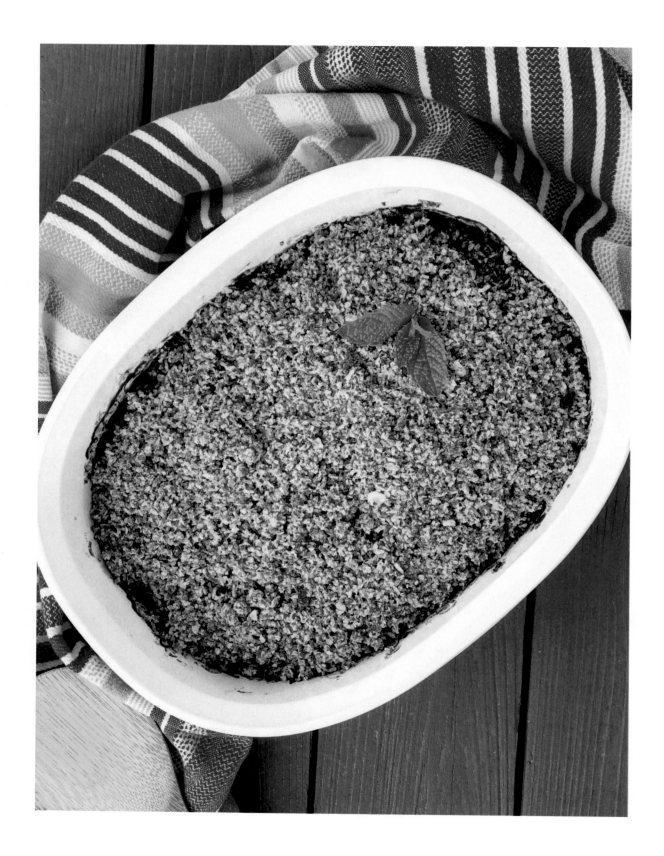

In a Pinch Blueberry Crisp

This super quick and easy blueberry crisp can be whipped up in minutes and enjoyed shortly after. We like to savour it on its own or pair it with whipped coconut cream or even a la mode, as it is hard to have a warm blueberry crisp or pie without any dairy-free ice cream.

Gluten-free   Ready in 45 minutes   Serves 6

¾ cup gluten-free rolled oats, finely ground
¼ cup shredded unsweetened coconut
¼ cup brown sugar
4 cups blueberries
1 tbsp brown sugar
1 tbsp lemon juice
1 tsp cinnamon
¼ cup coconut oil
pinch of sea salt

Preheat oven to 375°F. Grease a 9 x 11 baking dish.

Place blueberries in a large bowl and pour lemon juice and 1 tbsp brown sugar over them. Mix together.

Pour blueberry mixture into the baking dish.

Prepare crumble top. Pulse rolled oats in a mini chop so it makes an oat flour. In a bowl, mix rolled oats, sugar, cinnamon, coconut, sea salt, and coconut oil. Sprinkle over top of the blueberries in the baking dish.

Bake for 35 minutes.

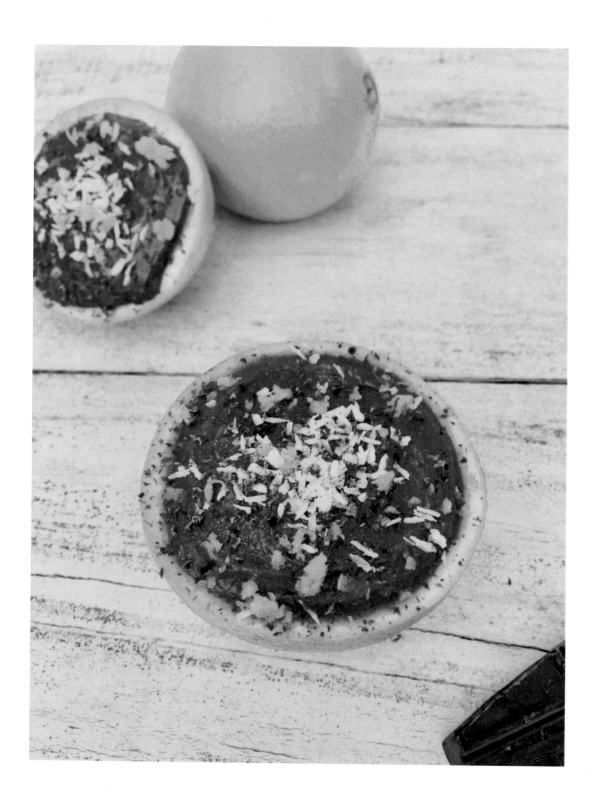

Orange Chocolate Avocado Pudding

This quick chocolate pudding is almost an instant pudding because it comes together with such ease. It is light and velvety for a perfect after lunch or dinner dessert. This a great way to incorporate healthy fats into sweets.

Gluten-free   Ready in 10 minutes   Serves 3

2 avocados
3 tbsp maple syrup
4 tbsp cocoa powder
1 tbsp almond milk
2 tbsp orange juice
½ zest of an orange
Pinch of sea salt

Cut avocados in half, remove pits, and scoop into a medium bowl.

Sift in cocoa and combine all other ingredients into the bowl. With a stick blender, purée. Set in fridge to chill and or serve right away.

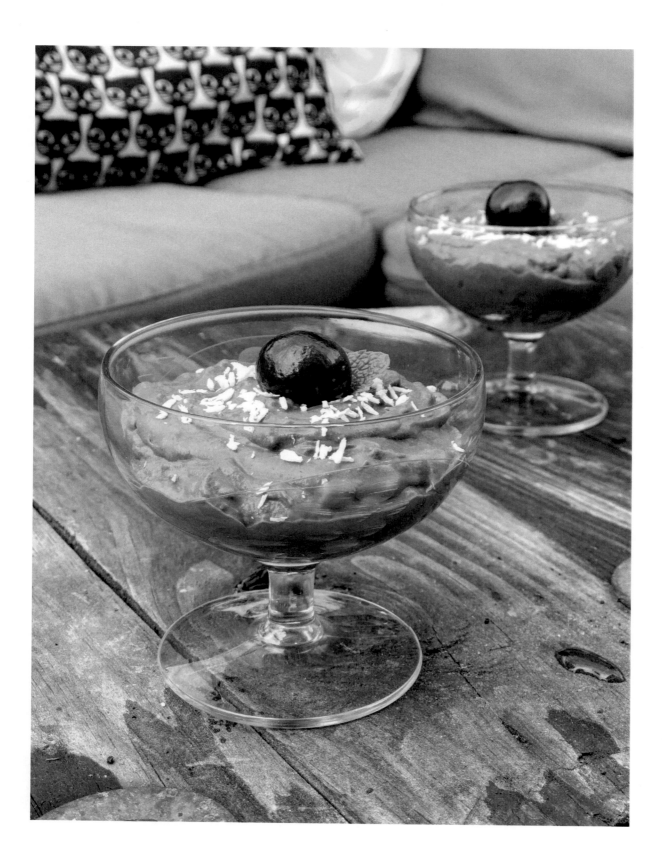

Coconut & Chocolate Mousse

Sometimes the best dessert is a simple, light chocolate mousse. This coconut and chocolate mousse has such a light and airy feel that it complements a warm summer meal superbly.

Gluten-free   Ready in 10 minutes   Serves 3

1 avocado
200 ml coconut milk
4 tbsp cocoa
4 tbsp maple syrup
1 tbsp chia seed
shredded coconut for garnish (optional)

In a medium mixing bowl, scoop in avocados (removing the pits). Add coconut milk, cocoa powder, and maple syrup and with a stick blender, purée.

Fold in 1 tbsp of chia seeds and top with shredded coconut. Serve and enjoy.

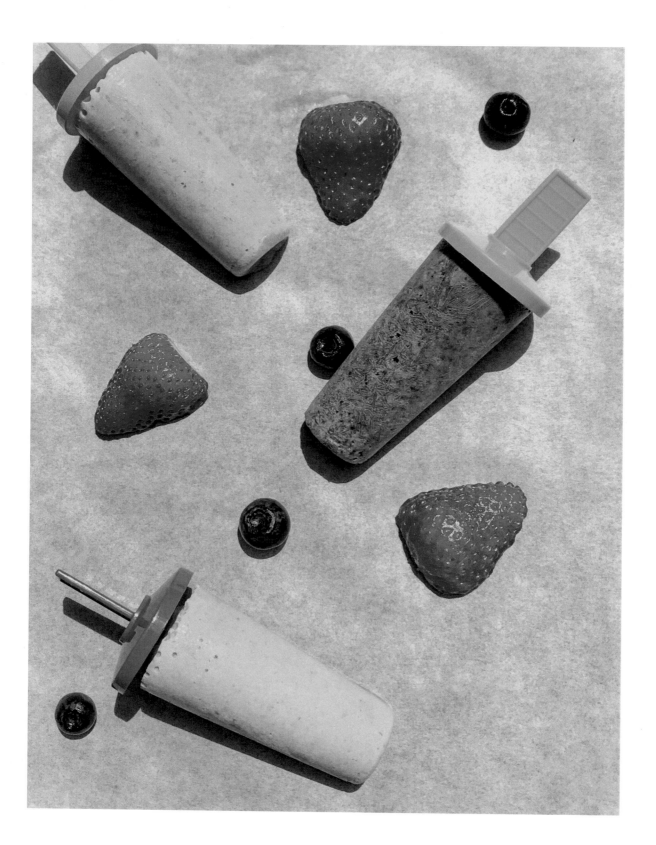

Frozen Summer Berry Yogurt Popsicles

Beat the summer heat with this healthy treat! Having frozen yogurt popsicles hidden in the freezer helps us stay cool after afternoon activities. Making our own frozen treats allows us to stay health-conscious by keeping them sugar-free.

Gluten-free   Ready in 5-6 hours   Makes 6 popsicles

1 cup vegan yogurt
¾ cup fruit of your choice (I made strawberry
**   and blueberry)**
¼ cup non-dairy milk

Place all ingredients in the blender and purée.

Pour yogurt mixture into popsicle containers and freeze for about 5-6 hours.

Once frozen, serve and enjoy.

Nutritional Breakdowns of Recipes

Rise and Shine

Coconut Kale & Banana Smoothie

Total	Item Name Coconut Kale & Banana Smoothie
1	Quantity
Serving	Measure
748.26	Cals (kcal)
11.4	Prot (g)
22.99	Carb (g)
3.02	TotFib (g)
0.12	TotSolFib (g)
7.72	Sugar (g)
3.52	SugAdd (g)
73.75	Fat (g)
59.65	SatFat (g)
5.15	MonoFat (g)
4.56	PolyFat (g)
0	TransFat (g)
0	Chol (mg)
976.97	Vit A-IU (IU)
42.64	Vit A-RAE (mcg)
85.29	Caroten (mcg)
0	Retinol (mcg)
497.93	BetaCaro (mcg)
0.2	Vit B1 (mg)
0.21	Vit B2 (mg)
3.31	Vit B3 (mg)
4.99	Vit B3-NE (mg)
0.32	Vit B6 (mg)

0.75	Vit B12 (mcg)
1.42	Biot (mcg)
17.69	Vit C (mg)
30	Vit D-IU (IU)
0.75	Vit D-mcg (mcg)
0.6	Vit E-a-Toco (mg)
100.62	Folate (mcg)
61.27	Vit K (mcg)
0.83	Panto (mg)
151.92	Calc (mg)
0.23	Chrom (mcg)
0.99	Copp (mg)
0	Fluor (mg)
2.7	Iodine (mcg)
11.42	Iron (mg)
222.15	Magn (mg)
3.11	Mang (mg)
0.4	Moly (mcg)
470.15	Phos (mg)
1089.94	Pot (mg)
0.52	Sel (mcg)
63.17	Sod (mg)
2.69	Zinc (mg)
0.84	Omega3 (g)
3.09	Omega6 (g)
32.47	Chln (mg)

Mango-Pineapple Smoothie

Total	Item Name Mango-Pineapple Smoothie
1	Quantity
Serving	Measure
200.02	Cals (kcal)
7.37	Prot (g)
30.99	Carb (g)
6.39	TotFib (g)
0.56	TotSolFib (g)
21.58	Sugar (g)
0	SugAdd (g)
5.92	Fat (g)
0.7	SatFat (g)
1.09	MonoFat (g)
3.88	PolyFat (g)
0.01	TransFat (g)
0	Chol (mg)
2024.52	Vit A-IU (IU)
88.73	Vit A-RAE (mcg)
177.45	Caroten (mcg)
0	Retinol (mcg)
832.39	BetaCaro (mcg)
0.17	Vit B1 (mg)
0.33	Vit B2 (mg)
1.42	Vit B3 (mg)
2.29	Vit B3-NE (mg)
0.17	Vit B6 (mg)
1.51	Vit B12 (mcg)
0.13	Biot (mcg)
70.57	Vit C (mg)
60	Vit D-IU (IU)
1.5	Vit D-mcg (mcg)
4.01	Vit E-a-Toco (mg)
97.02	Folate (mcg)
40.35	Vit K (mcg)
0.3	Panto (mg)
237.67	Calc (mg)
--	Chrom (mcg)
0.26	Copp (mg)
--	Fluor (mg)
0.15	Iodine (mcg)
1.91	Iron (mg)
82.22	Magn (mg)
0.89	Mang (mg)
0.37	Moly (mcg)
164.6	Phos (mg)
553.32	Pot (mg)
4.75	Sel (mcg)
48.86	Sod (mg)
0.68	Zinc (mg)
1.82	Omega3 (g)
0.8	Omega6 (g)
11.17	Chln (mg)

Raspberry-Banana Smoothie

Total	Item Name Raspberry-Banana Smoothie
1	Quantity
Serving	Measure
190.51	Cals (kcal)
7.22	Prot (g)
22.38	Carb (g)
7.63	TotFib (g)
0.03	TotSolFib (g)
10.75	Sugar (g)
0	SugAdd (g)
8.85	Fat (g)
1.02	SatFat (g)
2.73	MonoFat (g)
4.51	PolyFat (g)
0	TransFat (g)
0	Chol (mg)
387.42	Vit A-IU (IU)
7.82	Vit A-RAE (mcg)
13.79	Caroten (mcg)
0	Retinol (mcg)
40.07	BetaCaro (mcg)
0.19	Vit B1 (mg)
0.37	Vit B2 (mg)
1.75	Vit B3 (mg)
2.32	Vit B3-NE (mg)
0.27	Vit B6 (mg)
1.5	Vit B12 (mcg)
1.61	Biot (mcg)
39.54	Vit C (mg)
60	Vit D-IU (IU)
1.5	Vit D-mcg (mcg)
0.7	Vit E-a-Toco (mg)
75.83	Folate (mcg)
6.96	Vit K (mcg)
0.61	Panto (mg)
187.83	Calc (mg)
0.65	Chrom (mcg)
0.24	Copp (mg)
0	Fluor (mg)
3.63	Iodine (mcg)
1.71	Iron (mg)
98.73	Magn (mg)
0.75	Mang (mg)
--	Moly (mcg)
197.46	Phos (mg)
623.99	Pot (mg)
1.3	Sel (mcg)
40.27	Sod (mg)
1.05	Zinc (mg)
1.36	Omega3 (g)
1.89	Omega6 (g)
15.33	Chln (mg)

Peanut Butter Smoothie

Total	Item Name Peanut Butter Smoothie
1	Quantity
Serving	Measure
293.68	Cals (kcal)
12.66	Prot (g)
14.67	Carb (g)
5.09	TotFib (g)
0.5	TotSolFib (g)
5.75	Sugar (g)
0.46	SugAdd (g)
22.19	Fat (g)
2.97	SatFat (g)
5.72	MonoFat (g)
12.5	PolyFat (g)
0.01	TransFat (g)
0	Chol (mg)
398.13	Vit A-IU (IU)
1.16	Vit A-RAE (mcg)
2.31	Caroten (mcg)
0	Retinol (mcg)
10.16	BetaCaro (mcg)
0.15	Vit B1 (mg)
0.46	Vit B2 (mg)
1.92	Vit B3 (mg)
3.51	Vit B3-NE (mg)
0.25	Vit B6 (mg)
2.25	Vit B12 (mcg)
11.07	Biot (mcg)
2.93	Vit C (mg)
90	Vit D-IU (IU)
2.25	Vit D-mcg (mcg)
1.05	Vit E-a-Toco (mg)
79.94	Folate (mcg)
1.31	Vit K (mcg)
0.37	Panto (mg)
257.42	Calc (mg)
0.54	Chrom (mcg)
0.44	Copp (mg)
0	Fluor (mg)
3.68	Iodine (mcg)
2.36	Iron (mg)
136.03	Magn (mg)
1.17	Mang (mg)
4.31	Moly (mcg)
280.85	Phos (mg)
563.55	Pot (mg)
2.99	Sel (mcg)
56.07	Sod (mg)
1.48	Zinc (mg)
2.15	Omega3 (g)
8.45	Omega6 (g)
21.5	Chln (mg)

Cha Cha-Chai-Chia Seed Pudding

Total	Item Name Cha Cha-Chai-Chia Seed Pudding
1	Quantity
Serving	Measure
181.74	Cals (kcal)
8.12	Prot (g)
17.41	Carb (g)
8.46	TotFib (g)
--	TotSolFib (g)
5.34	Sugar (g)
0	SugAdd (g)
9.21	Fat (g)
1.13	SatFat (g)
0.5	MonoFat (g)
4.98	PolyFat (g)
0.03	TransFat (g)
0	Chol (mg)
393.64	Vit A-IU (IU)
0.68	Vit A-RAE (mcg)
1.36	Caroten (mcg)
0	Retinol (mcg)
0.84	BetaCaro (mcg)
0.13	Vit B1 (mg)
0.42	Vit B2 (mg)
1.89	Vit B3 (mg)
3.2	Vit B3-NE (mg)
0	Vit B6 (mg)
2.27	Vit B12 (mcg)
--	Biot (mcg)
0.42	Vit C (mg)
90.41	Vit D-IU (IU)
2.21	Vit D-mcg (mcg)
0.13	Vit E-a-Toco (mg)
28.93	Folate (mcg)
0.3	Vit K (mcg)
0	Panto (mg)
367.84	Calc (mg)
--	Chrom (mcg)
0.2	Copp (mg)
--	Fluor (mg)
--	Iodine (mcg)
2.58	Iron (mg)
101.74	Magn (mg)
0.87	Mang (mg)
--	Moly (mcg)
182.2	Phos (mg)
322.12	Pot (mg)
15.99	Sel (mcg)
75.69	Sod (mg)
1.47	Zinc (mg)
3.75	Omega3 (g)
1.23	Omega6 (g)
0.2	Chln (mg)

Goji Berry Granola & Yogurt

Total	Item Name Goji Berry Granola & Yogurt
1	Quantity
Serving = ¼ cup of granola and 150 grams of yogurt	Measure
309.65	Cals (kcal)
7.61	Prot (g)
41.98	Carb (g)
4.18	TotFib (g)
0.55	TotSolFib (g)
24	Sugar (g)
3.69	SugAdd (g)
13.11	Fat (g)
5.92	SatFat (g)
2.59	MonoFat (g)
1.45	PolyFat (g)
0	TransFat (g)
0	Chol (mg)
617.23	Vit A-IU (IU)
30.87	Vit A-RAE (mcg)
61.72	Caroten (mcg)
0	Retinol (mcg)
0.53	BetaCaro (mcg)
0.03	Vit B1 (mg)
0.15	Vit B2 (mg)
0.4	Vit B3 (mg)
0.92	Vit B3-NE (mg)
0.03	Vit B6 (mg)
0	Vit B12 (mcg)
--	Biot (mcg)

27.65	Vit C (mg)
0	Vit D-IU (IU)
0	Vit D-mcg (mcg)
1.5	Vit E-a-Toco (mg)
4.78	Folate (mcg)
0.32	Vit K (mcg)
0.09	Panto (mg)
297.42	Calc (mg)
0	Chrom (mcg)
0.14	Copp (mg)
0	Fluor (mg)
3.98	Iodine (mcg)
2.18	Iron (mg)
54.67	Magn (mg)
0.56	Mang (mg)
0	Moly (mcg)
118.5	Phos (mg)
146.27	Pot (mg)
1.39	Sel (mcg)
46.63	Sod (mg)
0.81	Zinc (mg)
0	Omega3 (g)
1.45	Omega6 (g)
5.98	Chln (mg)

Peaches 'n' Cream Oatmeal

Total	Item Name Peaches 'n' Cream Oatmeal
1	Quantity
Serving	Measure
230.71	Cals (kcal)
9.16	Prot (g)
30.84	Carb (g)
6.7	TotFib (g)
0.65	TotSolFib (g)
9.11	Sugar (g)
2.28	SugAdd (g)
8.68	Fat (g)
1.05	SatFat (g)
1.04	MonoFat (g)
5.05	PolyFat (g)
0.01	TransFat (g)
0	Chol (mg)
415.03	Vit A-IU (IU)
12.44	Vit A-RAE (mcg)
24.88	Caroten (mcg)
0	Retinol (mcg)
122.03	BetaCaro (mcg)
0.17	Vit B1 (mg)
0.22	Vit B2 (mg)
1.64	Vit B3 (mg)
2.53	Vit B3-NE (mg)
0.07	Vit B6 (mg)
1	Vit B12 (mcg)
0.15	Biot (mcg)
5.09	Vit C (mg)
40	Vit D-IU (IU)

Total	Item Name
1	Vit D-mcg (mcg)
0.63	Vit E-a-Toco (mg)
34.13	Folate (mcg)
2.15	Vit K (mcg)
0.15	Panto (mg)
160.74	Calc (mg)
--	Chrom (mcg)
0.22	Copp (mg)
0	Fluor (mg)
2.25	Iodine (mcg)
2.61	Iron (mg)
122.05	Magn (mg)
0.69	Mang (mg)
--	Moly (mcg)
297.22	Phos (mg)
455.82	Pot (mg)
3.87	Sel (mcg)
25.56	Sod (mg)
1.59	Zinc (mg)
2.27	Omega3 (g)
1.95	Omega6 (g)
7.35	Chln (mg)

Blueberry Oatmeal

Total	Item Name Blueberry Oatmeal
1	Quantity
Serving	Measure
213.37	Cals (kcal)
8.75	Prot (g)
26.76	Carb (g)
6.5	TotFib (g)
0.75	TotSolFib (g)
4.44	Sugar (g)
0	SugAdd (g)
8.62	Fat (g)
1.05	SatFat (g)
1.01	MonoFat (g)
5.04	PolyFat (g)
0.01	TransFat (g)
0	Chol (mg)
190.51	Vit A-IU (IU)
1.21	Vit A-RAE (mcg)
2.43	Caroten (mcg)
0	Retinol (mcg)
12.37	BetaCaro (mcg)
0.17	Vit B1 (mg)
0.21	Vit B2 (mg)
1.19	Vit B3 (mg)
1.98	Vit B3-NE (mg)
0.07	Vit B6 (mg)
1	Vit B12 (mcg)
--	Biot (mcg)
3.73	Vit C (mg)
40	Vit D-IU (IU)
1	Vit D-mcg (mcg)

0.29	Vit E-a-Toco (mg)
33.35	Folate (mcg)
7.34	Vit K (mcg)
0.08	Panto (mg)
158.18	Calc (mg)
--	Chrom (mcg)
0.19	Copp (mg)
--	Fluor (mg)
--	Iodine (mcg)
2.51	Iron (mg)
117.48	Magn (mg)
0.76	Mang (mg)
--	Moly (mcg)
286.64	Phos (mg)
341.15	Pot (mg)
3.83	Sel (mcg)
25.86	Sod (mg)
1.52	Zinc (mg)
2.29	Omega3 (g)
1.92	Omega6 (g)
4.99	Chln (mg)

Maple-Nut Granola Bars

Total	Item Name Maple-Nut Granola Bars
1	Quantity
Serving	Measure
272.55	Cals (kcal)
6.48	Prot (g)
20.45	Carb (g)
4.04	TotFib (g)
0.6	TotSolFib (g)
8.14	Sugar (g)
6.73	SugAdd (g)
19.55	Fat (g)
7.57	SatFat (g)
5.46	MonoFat (g)
4.87	PolyFat (g)
0.01	TransFat (g)
0	Chol (mg)
0.97	Vit A-IU (IU)
0.05	Vit A-RAE (mcg)
0.1	Caroten (mcg)
0	Retinol (mcg)
0.57	BetaCaro (mcg)
0.11	Vit B1 (mg)
0.22	Vit B2 (mg)
1.92	Vit B3 (mg)
2.83	Vit B3-NE (mg)
0.11	Vit B6 (mg)
0	Vit B12 (mcg)
11.97	Biot (mcg)
0.15	Vit C (mg)
0	Vit D-IU (IU)

Total	Item Name
0	Vit D-mcg (mcg)
2.29	Vit E-a-Toco (mg)
19.47	Folate (mcg)
0.35	Vit K (mcg)
0.25	Panto (mg)
47.76	Calc (mg)
0.46	Chrom (mcg)
0.24	Copp (mg)
0.01	Fluor (mg)
12.98	Iodine (mcg)
1.32	Iron (mg)
73.89	Magn (mg)
0.89	Mang (mg)
1.08	Moly (mcg)
150.19	Phos (mg)
233.93	Pot (mg)
2.67	Sel (mcg)
53.83	Sod (mg)
1.13	Zinc (mg)
1.13	Omega3 (g)
3.71	Omega6 (g)
15.18	Chln (mg)

High-Energy Bites Carrot Cake

Total	Item Name HE Bites Carrot Cake
1	Quantity
Serving	Measure
96.71	Cals (kcal)
2.18	Prot (g)
6.79	Carb (g)
1.8	TotFib (g)
0.45	TotSolFib (g)
0.85	Sugar (g)
0	SugAdd (g)
7.35	Fat (g)
2.45	SatFat (g)
0.75	MonoFat (g)
3.48	PolyFat (g)
0	TransFat (g)
0	Chol (mg)
1150.54	Vit A-IU (IU)
57.53	Vit A-RAE (mcg)
115.05	Caroten (mcg)
0	Retinol (mcg)
570.68	BetaCaro (mcg)
0.03	Vit B1 (mg)
0.02	Vit B2 (mg)
0.18	Vit B3 (mg)
0.43	Vit B3-NE (mg)
0.06	Vit B6 (mg)
0	Vit B12 (mcg)
1.41	Biot (mcg)
0.56	Vit C (mg)
0	Vit D-IU (IU)
0	Vit D-mcg (mcg)
0.11	Vit E-a-Toco (mg)
8.8	Folate (mcg)
1.17	Vit K (mcg)
0.09	Panto (mg)
14.36	Calc (mg)
0.03	Chrom (mcg)
0.15	Copp (mg)
0	Fluor (mg)
3.88	Iodine (mcg)
0.63	Iron (mg)
24.52	Magn (mg)
0.4	Mang (mg)
2.5	Moly (mcg)
59.48	Phos (mg)
96.27	Pot (mg)
1.02	Sel (mcg)
18.11	Sod (mg)
0.46	Zinc (mg)
0.66	Omega3 (g)
2.82	Omega6 (g)
4.25	Chln (mg)

High-Energy Bites Lemon Zinger

Total	Item Name HE Bites Lemon Zinger
1	Quantity
Serving	Measure
98.45	Cals (kcal)
2.88	Prot (g)
6.86	Carb (g)
1.85	TotFib (g)
0.21	TotSolFib (g)
0.58	Sugar (g)
0	SugAdd (g)
7.2	Fat (g)
2.39	SatFat (g)
1.76	MonoFat (g)
2.11	PolyFat (g)
0	TransFat (g)
0	Chol (mg)
5.61	Vit A-IU (IU)
0.28	Vit A-RAE (mcg)
0.56	Caroten (mcg)
0	Retinol (mcg)
2.74	BetaCaro (mcg)
0.14	Vit B1 (mg)
0.04	Vit B2 (mg)
0.77	Vit B3 (mg)
1.25	Vit B3-NE (mg)
0.13	Vit B6 (mg)
0	Vit B12 (mcg)
0	Biot (mcg)
0.66	Vit C (mg)
0	Vit D-IU (IU)

0	Vit D-mcg (mcg)
3.19	Vit E-a-Toco (mg)
20.81	Folate (mcg)
0.02	Vit K (mcg)
0.13	Panto (mg)
10.97	Calc (mg)
0	Chrom (mcg)
0.19	Copp (mg)
0.01	Fluor (mg)
6.35	Iodine (mcg)
0.88	Iron (mg)
41.36	Magn (mg)
0.28	Mang (mg)
0	Moly (mcg)
91.22	Phos (mg)
100.74	Pot (mg)
5.4	Sel (mcg)
26	Sod (mg)
0.66	Zinc (mg)
0.01	Omega3 (g)
2.1	Omega6 (g)
5.77	Chln (mg)

Never "Blue"berry Oatmeal Muffins

Total	Item Name Never "Blue"berry Oatmeal Muffins
1	Quantity
Serving	Measure
179.6	Cals (kcal)
3.38	Prot (g)
27.5	Carb (g)
3.37	TotFib (g)
0.17	TotSolFib (g)
11.68	Sugar (g)
9.13	SugAdd (g)
6.06	Fat (g)
3.88	SatFat (g)
0.45	MonoFat (g)
0.59	PolyFat (g)
0	TransFat (g)
0	Chol (mg)
44.2	Vit A-IU (IU)
0.65	Vit A-RAE (mcg)
1.3	Caroten (mcg)
0	Retinol (mcg)
6.5	BetaCaro (mcg)
0.03	Vit B1 (mg)
0.05	Vit B2 (mg)
0.15	Vit B3 (mg)
0.23	Vit B3-NE (mg)
0.05	Vit B6 (mg)
0.19	Vit B12 (mcg)
0.26	Biot (mcg)
2.06	Vit C (mg)
7.5	Vit D-IU (IU)
0.19	Vit D-mcg (mcg)
0.09	Vit E-a-Toco (mg)
7.47	Folate (mcg)
2.51	Vit K (mcg)
0.06	Panto (mg)
25.73	Calc (mg)
0.08	Chrom (mcg)
0.03	Copp (mg)
0	Fluor (mg)
4.95	Iodine (mcg)
1.14	Iron (mg)
15.58	Magn (mg)
0.1	Mang (mg)
0	Moly (mcg)
31.96	Phos (mg)
91.37	Pot (mg)
0.41	Sel (mcg)
231.42	Sod (mg)
0.23	Zinc (mg)
0.28	Omega3 (g)
0.16	Omega6 (g)
2.64	Chln (mg)

Banana Coconut Chocolate Chip Pancakes

Total	Item Name Banana Coconut Chocolate Chip Pancakes
1	Quantity
Serving	Measure
284.51	Cals (kcal)
5.67	Prot (g)
30.13	Carb (g)
6.38	TotFib (g)
0.04	TotSolFib (g)
9.02	Sugar (g)
0	SugAdd (g)
16.13	Fat (g)
10.43	SatFat (g)
0.82	MonoFat (g)
1.63	PolyFat (g)
0.01	TransFat (g)
0	Chol (mg)
76.98	Vit A-IU (IU)
0.72	Vit A-RAE (mcg)
1.45	Caroten (mcg)
0	Retinol (mcg)
5.11	BetaCaro (mcg)
0.05	Vit B1 (mg)
0.09	Vit B2 (mg)
0.5	Vit B3 (mg)
0.84	Vit B3-NE (mg)
0.09	Vit B6 (mg)
0.38	Vit B12 (mcg)
0.51	Biot (mcg)
1.82	Vit C (mg)
15	Vit D-IU (IU)

0.38	Vit D-mcg (mcg)
0.06	Vit E-a-Toco (mg)
14.46	Folate (mcg)
0.2	Vit K (mcg)
0.1	Panto (mg)
82.59	Calc (mg)
0.16	Chrom (mcg)
0.09	Copp (mg)
0.01	Fluor (mg)
10.01	Iodine (mcg)
2.56	Iron (mg)
29.62	Magn (mg)
0.27	Mang (mg)
0	Moly (mcg)
61.28	Phos (mg)
155.03	Pot (mg)
3.04	Sel (mcg)
148.52	Sod (mg)
0.31	Zinc (mg)
0.9	Omega3 (g)
0.42	Omega6 (g)
3.6	Chln (mg)

French Toast with Glazed Peaches & Cherry Compote

Total	Item Name French Toast with Glazed Peaches & Cherry Compote
1	Quantity
Serving	Measure
1068.38	Cals (kcal)
34.97	Prot (g)
191.75	Carb (g)
12.11	TotFib (g)
1.96	TotSolFib (g)
46.45	Sugar (g)
12.55	SugAdd (g)
19.81	Fat (g)
9.38	SatFat (g)
2.35	MonoFat (g)
4.83	PolyFat (g)
0.02	TransFat (g)
0	Chol (mg)
533.57	Vit A-IU (IU)
18.35	Vit A-RAE (mcg)
36.69	Caroten (mcg)
0	Retinol (mcg)
177.47	BetaCaro (mcg)
2.1	Vit B1 (mg)
1.61	Vit B2 (mg)
14.75	Vit B3 (mg)
15.22	Vit B3-NE (mg)
0.56	Vit B6 (mg)
1	Vit B12 (mcg)
4.65	Biot (mcg)
13.37	Vit C (mg)

40	Vit D-IU (IU)
1	Vit D-mcg (mcg)
1.4	Vit E-a-Toco (mg)
381.84	Folate (mcg)
5.13	Vit K (mcg)
1.66	Panto (mg)
288.44	Calc (mg)
0.47	Chrom (mcg)
0.6	Copp (mg)
0.01	Fluor (mg)
22.79	Iodine (mcg)
11.95	Iron (mg)
148.58	Magn (mg)
2.27	Mang (mg)
--	Moly (mcg)
388.5	Phos (mg)
909.74	Pot (mg)
81.41	Sel (mcg)
1700.32	Sod (mg)
3.45	Zinc (mg)
1.26	Omega3 (g)
2.74	Omega6 (g)
37.84	Chln (mg)

Patatas Bravas with Tempeh & Roasted Garlic Kale

Total	Item Name Patatas Bravas with Tempeh & Roasted Garlic Kale		
1	Quantity	0	Vit D-IU (IU)
Serving	Measure	0	Vit D-mcg (mcg)
547.92	Cals (kcal)	0.37	Vit E-a-Toco (mg)
14.6	Prot (g)	69.85	Folate (mcg)
44.78	Carb (g)	66.69	Vit K (mcg)
7.41	TotFib (g)	0.8	Panto (mg)
0.12	TotSolFib (g)	94.21	Calc (mg)
4.85	Sugar (g)	0.26	Chrom (mcg)
0	SugAdd (g)	0.68	Copp (mg)
37.26	Fat (g)	0.02	Fluor (mg)
5.25	SatFat (g)	17.07	Iodine (mcg)
21.14	MonoFat (g)	3.03	Iron (mg)
5.8	PolyFat (g)	92.05	Magn (mg)
0	TransFat (g)	1.01	Mang (mg)
0	Chol (mg)	3.3	Moly (mcg)
1150.83	Vit A-IU (IU)	268.9	Phos (mg)
57.54	Vit A-RAE (mcg)	1316.93	Pot (mg)
115.08	Caroten (mcg)	1.53	Sel (mcg)
0	Retinol (mcg)	112.24	Sod (mg)
665.22	BetaCaro (mcg)	1.36	Zinc (mg)
0.24	Vit B1 (mg)	0.42	Omega3 (g)
0.24	Vit B2 (mg)	5.37	Omega6 (g)
3.92	Vit B3 (mg)	39.39	Chln (mg)
6.08	Vit B3-NE (mg)		
0.56	Vit B6 (mg)		
0.03	Vit B12 (mcg)		
2.25	Biot (mcg)		
38.04	Vit C (mg)		

"Bacon & Egg" Skillet

Total	Item Name "Bacon & Egg" Skillet
1	Quantity
Serving	Measure
276.96	Cals (kcal)
12.81	Prot (g)
40.45	Carb (g)
5.11	TotFib (g)
0	TotSolFib (g)
4.27	Sugar (g)
0	SugAdd (g)
8.33	Fat (g)
1.22	SatFat (g)
4.01	MonoFat (g)
2.61	PolyFat (g)
0	TransFat (g)
0	Chol (mg)
583.21	Vit A-IU (IU)
29.16	Vit A-RAE (mcg)
58.32	Caroten (mcg)
0	Retinol (mcg)
311.6	BetaCaro (mcg)
0.96	Vit B1 (mg)
0.87	Vit B2 (mg)
6.88	Vit B3 (mg)
8.4	Vit B3-NE (mg)
0.86	Vit B6 (mg)
1.14	Vit B12 (mcg)
1.1	Biot (mcg)
38.28	Vit C (mg)
0.75	Vit D-IU (IU)

Total	Item Name
0.02	Vit D-mcg (mcg)
0.29	Vit E-a-Toco (mg)
57.39	Folate (mcg)
8.12	Vit K (mcg)
1.09	Panto (mg)
109.67	Calc (mg)
0	Chrom (mcg)
0.52	Copp (mg)
0.03	Fluor (mg)
25.29	Iodine (mcg)
3.24	Iron (mg)
68.52	Magn (mg)
0.72	Mang (mg)
1.09	Moly (mcg)
222.61	Phos (mg)
1230.79	Pot (mg)
7.85	Sel (mcg)
142.28	Sod (mg)
1.4	Zinc (mg)
0.12	Omega3 (g)
1.31	Omega6 (g)
42.42	Chln (mg)

Breakfast Burrito

Total	Item Name Breakfast Burrito
1	Quantity
Serving	Measure
463.79	Cals (kcal)
18.58	Prot (g)
68.89	Carb (g)
10.04	TotFib (g)
1.26	TotSolFib (g)
6.66	Sugar (g)
0	SugAdd (g)
14.35	Fat (g)
3.46	SatFat (g)
2.28	MonoFat (g)
1.77	PolyFat (g)
0	TransFat (g)
0	Chol (mg)
800.07	Vit A-IU (IU)
40	Vit A-RAE (mcg)
80.01	Caroten (mcg)
0	Retinol (mcg)
429.06	BetaCaro (mcg)
0.74	Vit B1 (mg)
0.65	Vit B2 (mg)
4.05	Vit B3 (mg)
5.84	Vit B3-NE (mg)
0.53	Vit B6 (mg)
0.76	Vit B12 (mcg)
2.92	Biot (mcg)
23.73	Vit C (mg)
0.8	Vit D-IU (IU)
0.03	Vit D-mcg (mcg)

0.85	Vit E-a-Toco (mg)
137.59	Folate (mcg)
5.88	Vit K (mcg)
0.79	Panto (mg)
85.33	Calc (mg)
0.36	Chrom (mcg)
0.42	Copp (mg)
0.02	Fluor (mg)
16.95	Iodine (mcg)
3.45	Iron (mg)
72.13	Magn (mg)
0.76	Mang (mg)
3.48	Moly (mcg)
216.78	Phos (mg)
722.18	Pot (mg)
9.15	Sel (mcg)
735.43	Sod (mg)
1.62	Zinc (mg)
0.15	Omega3 (g)
0.83	Omega6 (g)
36.06	Chln (mg)

"You Gotta, Try This" Frittata

Total	Item Name "You Gotta, Try This" Frittata
1	Quantity
Serving	Measure
129.48	Cals (kcal)
9.24	Prot (g)
7.91	Carb (g)
1.82	TotFib (g)
0	TotSolFib (g)
2.33	Sugar (g)
0	SugAdd (g)
7.95	Fat (g)
1.07	SatFat (g)
3.46	MonoFat (g)
2.91	PolyFat (g)
0	TransFat (g)
0	Chol (mg)
570.14	Vit A-IU (IU)
28.51	Vit A-RAE (mcg)
57.01	Caroten (mcg)
0	Retinol (mcg)
322.71	BetaCaro (mcg)
1.6	Vit B1 (mg)
1.39	Vit B2 (mg)
6.91	Vit B3 (mg)
9.06	Vit B3-NE (mg)
0.87	Vit B6 (mg)
2.21	Vit B12 (mcg)
2.05	Biot (mcg)
4.68	Vit C (mg)
0.54	Vit D-IU (IU)
0.02	Vit D-mcg (mcg)
0.43	Vit E-a-Toco (mg)
31.8	Folate (mcg)
27.42	Vit K (mcg)
0.46	Panto (mg)
349.22	Calc (mg)
0	Chrom (mcg)
0.37	Copp (mg)
0.01	Fluor (mg)
12.69	Iodine (mcg)
6.54	Iron (mg)
43.52	Magn (mg)
0.82	Mang (mg)
0.47	Moly (mcg)
142.47	Phos (mg)
375.71	Pot (mg)
13.58	Sel (mcg)
62.14	Sod (mg)
1.37	Zinc (mg)
0.32	Omega3 (g)
2.59	Omega6 (g)
8.6	Chln (mg)

Please Note, nutritional vaules of all recipes may vary depending on the type of ingredients used "Nutritional analysis from Food Processor® Nutrition and Fitness Software version 11.5, ©2018 ESHA Research, Inc."

Savoury Sides

Ginger & Miso Squash Soup

Total	Item Name Ginger & Miso Squash Soup
1	Quantity
Serving = 1 cup	Measure
126.81	Cals (kcal)
1.59	Prot (g)
11.92	Carb (g)
1.92	TotFib (g)
3.83	Sugar (g)
0	SugAdd (g)
9.32	Fat (g)
6.4	SatFat (g)
1.98	MonoFat (g)
0.49	PolyFat (g)
0	TransFat (g)
0	Chol (mg)
6214.68	Vit A-IU (IU)
310.73	Vit A-RAE (mcg)
621.47	Caroten (mcg)
0	Retinol (mcg)
2471.66	BetaCaro (mcg)
0.07	Vit B1 (mg)
0.02	Vit B2 (mg)
0.95	Vit B3 (mg)
1.27	Vit B3-NE (mg)
0.13	Vit B6 (mg)
0	Vit B12 (mcg)
0.49	Biot (mcg)
14.21	Vit C (mg)
0	Vit D-IU (IU)
0	Vit D-mcg (mcg)
0.88	Vit E-a-Toco (mg)
22.48	Folate (mcg)
1.58	Vit K (mcg)
0.31	Panto (mg)
39.21	Calc (mg)
0.19	Chrom (mcg)
0.13	Copp (mg)
0	Fluor (mg)
4.3	Iodine (mcg)
1.58	Iron (mg)
37.34	Magn (mg)
0.42	Mang (mg)
3.25	Moly (mcg)
57.37	Phos (mg)
316.1	Pot (mg)
0.5	Sel (mcg)
76.5	Sod (mg)
0.33	Zinc (mg)
0.02	Omega3 (g)
0.13	Omega6 (g)
5.13	Chln (mg)

Save Yourself Some Thyme Split Pea Soup

Total	Item Name Save Yourself Some Thyme Split Pea Soup
1	Quantity
Serving = 1 cup	Measure
110.44	Cals (kcal)
5.08	Prot (g)
20.16	Carb (g)
5.9	TotFib (g)
3.11	Sugar (g)
0	SugAdd (g)
1.44	Fat (g)
0.21	SatFat (g)
0.87	MonoFat (g)
0.25	PolyFat (g)
0	TransFat (g)
0	Chol (mg)
2763.61	Vit A-IU (IU)
138.18	Vit A-RAE (mcg)
276.36	Caroten (mcg)
0	Retinol (mcg)
1378.59	BetaCaro (mcg)
0.17	Vit B1 (mg)
0.07	Vit B2 (mg)
1.08	Vit B3 (mg)
2.03	Vit B3-NE (mg)
0.19	Vit B6 (mg)
0	Vit B12 (mcg)
0.53	Biot (mcg)
9.87	Vit C (mg)
0	Vit D-IU (IU)
0	Vit D-mcg (mcg)

0.33	Vit E-a-Toco (mg)
60.96	Folate (mcg)
12.5	Vit K (mcg)
0.49	Panto (mg)
28.62	Calc (mg)
0.1	Chrom (mcg)
0.19	Copp (mg)
0.01	Fluor (mg)
8.6	Iodine (mcg)
1.43	Iron (mg)
21.4	Magn (mg)
0.33	Mang (mg)
2.1	Moly (mcg)
86.57	Phos (mg)
393.99	Pot (mg)
1.03	Sel (mcg)
58.37	Sod (mg)
0.78	Zinc (mg)
0.03	Omega3 (g)
0.22	Omega6 (g)
23.16	Chln (mg)

Tomato, Kale, & Lentil Soup

Total	Item Name Tomato, Kale, & Lentil Soup
1	Quantity
Serving = 1 cup	Measure
165.47	Cals (kcal)
9.29	Prot (g)
28.44	Carb (g)
7.76	TotFib (g)
3.82	Sugar (g)
0	SugAdd (g)
2.32	Fat (g)
0.22	SatFat (g)
1.01	MonoFat (g)
0.24	PolyFat (g)
0	TransFat (g)
0	Chol (mg)
1055	Vit A-IU (IU)
52.75	Vit A-RAE (mcg)
105.5	Caroten (mcg)
0	Retinol (mcg)
421	BetaCaro (mcg)
0.07	Vit B1 (mg)
0.02	Vit B2 (mg)
0.14	Vit B3 (mg)
0.21	Vit B3-NE (mg)
0.06	Vit B6 (mg)
0	Vit B12 (mcg)
0.61	Biot (mcg)
19.45	Vit C (mg)
0	Vit D-IU (IU)
0	Vit D-mcg (mcg)
0.15	Vit E-a-Toco (mg)
17.74	Folate (mcg)
50.3	Vit K (mcg)
0.07	Panto (mg)
66.28	Calc (mg)
0.05	Chrom (mcg)
0.11	Copp (mg)
0	Fluor (mg)
0.32	Iodine (mcg)
2.43	Iron (mg)
6.7	Magn (mg)
0.1	Mang (mg)
1.88	Moly (mcg)
15.37	Phos (mg)
563.54	Pot (mg)
0.29	Sel (mcg)
29.44	Sod (mg)
0.09	Zinc (mg)
0.01	Omega3 (g)
0.03	Omega6 (g)
2.14	Chln (mg)

Charred Tomato Soup

Total	Item Name Charred Tomato Soup
1	Quantity
Serving = 1 cup	Measure
80.41	Cals (kcal)
2.09	Prot (g)
13.4	Carb (g)
4	TotFib (g)
6.64	Sugar (g)
0.57	SugAdd (g)
1.82	Fat (g)
0.22	SatFat (g)
1.24	MonoFat (g)
0.27	PolyFat (g)
0	TransFat (g)
0	Chol (mg)
2119.49	Vit A-IU (IU)
105.97	Vit A-RAE (mcg)
211.95	Caroten (mcg)
0	Retinol (mcg)
738.73	BetaCaro (mcg)
0.02	Vit B1 (mg)
0.02	Vit B2 (mg)
0.16	Vit B3 (mg)
0.24	Vit B3-NE (mg)
0.06	Vit B6 (mg)
0	Vit B12 (mcg)
0.52	Biot (mcg)
27.19	Vit C (mg)
0	Vit D-IU (IU)
0	Vit D-mcg (mcg)
0.1	Vit E-a-Toco (mg)
9.62	Folate (mcg)
10.33	Vit K (mcg)
0.08	Panto (mg)
82.24	Calc (mg)
0.07	Chrom (mcg)
0.02	Copp (mg)
0.01	Fluor (mg)
12.78	Iodine (mcg)
0.16	Iron (mg)
4.98	Magn (mg)
0.08	Mang (mg)
1.72	Moly (mcg)
12.86	Phos (mg)
483.14	Pot (mg)
0.35	Sel (mcg)
88.94	Sod (mg)
0.09	Zinc (mg)
0.02	Omega3 (g)
0.24	Omega6 (g)
2.81	Chln (mg)

Fall Squash & Lentil Salad

Total	Item Name Fall Squash & Lentil Salad
1	Quantity
Serving	Measure
475.9	Cals (kcal)
10.84	Prot (g)
37.31	Carb (g)
8.29	TotFib (g)
6.78	Sugar (g)
3	SugAdd (g)
33.16	Fat (g)
3.73	SatFat (g)
22.56	MonoFat (g)
4.38	PolyFat (g)
0	TransFat (g)
0	Chol (mg)
4536.18	Vit A-IU (IU)
226.81	Vit A-RAE (mcg)
453.62	Caroten (mcg)
0	Retinol (mcg)
1851.73	BetaCaro (mcg)
0.13	Vit B1 (mg)
0.11	Vit B2 (mg)
0.74	Vit B3 (mg)
0.9	Vit B3-NE (mg)
0.14	Vit B6 (mg)
0	Vit B12 (mcg)
0.05	Biot (mcg)
40.56	Vit C (mg)
0	Vit D-IU (IU)
0	Vit D-mcg (mcg)

0.83	Vit E-a-Toco (mg)
26.5	Folate (mcg)
17.56	Vit K (mcg)
0.26	Panto (mg)
48.75	Calc (mg)
0.1	Chrom (mcg)
0.04	Copp (mg)
--	Fluor (mg)
0.4	Iodine (mcg)
3.17	Iron (mg)
20.03	Magn (mg)
0.24	Mang (mg)
4.54	Moly (mcg)
25.21	Phos (mg)
625.35	Pot (mg)
0.26	Sel (mcg)
50.78	Sod (mg)
0.2	Zinc (mg)
0.35	Omega3 (g)
4.03	Omega6 (g)
3.43	Chln (mg)

Rainbow Radish, Apple, & Quinoa Salad

Total	Item Name Rainbow Radish, Apple, & Quinoa Salad
1	Quantity
Serving	Measure
369.66	Cals (kcal)
6.86	Prot (g)
38.86	Carb (g)
5.43	TotFib (g)
8.32	Sugar (g)
1	SugAdd (g)
21.41	Fat (g)
2.47	SatFat (g)
13.86	MonoFat (g)
3.94	PolyFat (g)
0	TransFat (g)
0	Chol (mg)
341.69	Vit A-IU (IU)
17.08	Vit A-RAE (mcg)
34.17	Caroten (mcg)
0	Retinol (mcg)
204.35	BetaCaro (mcg)
0.19	Vit B1 (mg)
0.19	Vit B2 (mg)
0.87	Vit B3 (mg)
2.15	Vit B3-NE (mg)
0.29	Vit B6 (mg)
0	Vit B12 (mcg)
0.28	Biot (mcg)
17.05	Vit C (mg)
0	Vit D-IU (IU)
0	Vit D-mcg (mcg)

1.19	Vit E-a-Toco (mg)
97.44	Folate (mcg)
15.95	Vit K (mcg)
0.44	Panto (mg)
41.8	Calc (mg)
0	Chrom (mcg)
0.29	Copp (mg)
0.03	Fluor (mg)
25.14	Iodine (mcg)
2.28	Iron (mg)
95.23	Magn (mg)
0.99	Mang (mg)
2.04	Moly (mcg)
214.64	Phos (mg)
420.58	Pot (mg)
3.97	Sel (mcg)
111.72	Sod (mg)
1.47	Zinc (mg)
0.32	Omega3 (g)
3.62	Omega6 (g)
37.24	Chln (mg)

Garden Basil Pesto Pasta with Sundried Tomatoes & Olives

Total	Item Name Garden Basil Pesto Pasta with Sundried Tomatoes & Olives
1	Quantity
Serving	Measure
533.98	Cals (kcal)
8.75	Prot (g)
39.77	Carb (g)
4.58	TotFib (g)
5.16	Sugar (g)
0	SugAdd (g)
40.46	Fat (g)
5.19	SatFat (g)
22.71	MonoFat (g)
11.18	PolyFat (g)
0	TransFat (g)
0	Chol (mg)
968.46	Vit A-IU (IU)
48.42	Vit A-RAE (mcg)
96.85	Caroten (mcg)
0	Retinol (mcg)
577.09	BetaCaro (mcg)
0.85	Vit B1 (mg)
0.69	Vit B2 (mg)
4.21	Vit B3 (mg)
4.92	Vit B3-NE (mg)
0.58	Vit B6 (mg)
1.1	Vit B12 (mcg)
3.66	Biot (mcg)
93.81	Vit C (mg)
0	Vit D-IU (IU)

0	Vit D-mcg (mcg)
0.51	Vit E-a-Toco (mg)
42.15	Folate (mcg)
62.16	Vit K (mcg)
0.36	Panto (mg)
69.18	Calc (mg)
0	Chrom (mcg)
0.48	Copp (mg)
0.03	Fluor (mg)
26.32	Iodine (mcg)
2.35	Iron (mg)
53.39	Magn (mg)
0.85	Mang (mg)
6.64	Moly (mcg)
102.91	Phos (mg)
464.67	Pot (mg)
1.43	Sel (mcg)
230.54	Sod (mg)
0.94	Zinc (mg)
1.38	Omega3 (g)
5.8	Omega6 (g)
16.53	Chln (mg)

Rice Paper Spring Rolls with Coconut Peanut Sauce

Total	Item Name Rice Paper Spring Rolls with Cocount Peanut Sauce
1	Quantity
Serving	Measure
192.32	Cals (kcal)
4.64	Prot (g)
18.25	Carb (g)
1.88	TotFib (g)
7.22	Sugar (g)
1.76	SugAdd (g)
12.37	Fat (g)
3.56	SatFat (g)
4.69	MonoFat (g)
3.3	PolyFat (g)
0.01	TransFat (g)
0	Chol (mg)
2901.05	Vit A-IU (IU)
145.05	Vit A-RAE (mcg)
290.11	Caroten (mcg)
0	Retinol (mcg)
1421.61	BetaCaro (mcg)
0.05	Vit B1 (mg)
0.06	Vit B2 (mg)
1.84	Vit B3 (mg)
2.37	Vit B3-NE (mg)
0.14	Vit B6 (mg)
0	Vit B12 (mcg)
10.2	Biot (mcg)
21.72	Vit C (mg)
0	Vit D-IU (IU)
0	Vit D-mcg (mcg)

Total	Item Name
1.36	Vit E-a-Toco (mg)
27.01	Folate (mcg)
14.25	Vit K (mcg)
0.29	Panto (mg)
27.49	Calc (mg)
0.46	Chrom (mcg)
0.11	Copp (mg)
0	Fluor (mg)
4.17	Iodine (mcg)
0.93	Iron (mg)
31.36	Magn (mg)
0.35	Mang (mg)
2.21	Moly (mcg)
62.68	Phos (mg)
233.87	Pot (mg)
0.8	Sel (mcg)
44.84	Sod (mg)
0.45	Zinc (mg)
0.04	Omega3 (g)
3.24	Omega6 (g)
14.66	Chln (mg)

Avocado Sushi Roll

Total	Item Name Avocado Sushi Roll
1	Quantity
Serving	Measure
348.64	Cals (kcal)
5.99	Prot (g)
72.8	Carb (g)
3.9	TotFib (g)
6.96	Sugar (g)
0	SugAdd (g)
3.29	Fat (g)
0.54	SatFat (g)
2	MonoFat (g)
0.47	PolyFat (g)
0	TransFat (g)
0	Chol (mg)
418.59	Vit A-IU (IU)
20.93	Vit A-RAE (mcg)
41.86	Caroten (mcg)
0	Retinol (mcg)
242.03	BetaCaro (mcg)
0.09	Vit B1 (mg)
0.1	Vit B2 (mg)
1.84	Vit B3 (mg)
2.99	Vit B3-NE (mg)
0.23	Vit B6 (mg)
0	Vit B12 (mcg)
0.79	Biot (mcg)
11.77	Vit C (mg)
0	Vit D-IU (IU)
0	Vit D-mcg (mcg)
0.73	Vit E-a-Toco (mg)

Total	Item Name
35.5	Folate (mcg)
8.29	Vit K (mcg)
1.38	Panto (mg)
11.01	Calc (mg)
--	Chrom (mcg)
0.24	Copp (mg)
0	Fluor (mg)
0.38	Iodine (mcg)
0.87	Iron (mg)
27.69	Magn (mg)
0.91	Mang (mg)
0.65	Moly (mcg)
93.4	Phos (mg)
215.66	Pot (mg)
12.43	Sel (mcg)
4.14	Sod (mg)
1.07	Zinc (mg)
0.06	Omega3 (g)
0.41	Omega6 (g)
6.03	Chln (mg)

Please note the iodine vaule for nori was unavailable, therefore the amount would be higher then the listed value

Lemon Cumin Hummus

Total	Item Name Lemon Cumin Hummus
1	Quantity
Serving = 1/4 cup	Measure
225.13	Cals (kcal)
5.28	Prot (g)
14.25	Carb (g)
2.73	TotFib (g)
2.18	Sugar (g)
0	SugAdd (g)
17.19	Fat (g)
2	SatFat (g)
10.01	MonoFat (g)
4.45	PolyFat (g)
0.02	TransFat (g)
0	Chol (mg)
51.75	Vit A-IU (IU)
2.59	Vit A-RAE (mcg)
5.18	Caroten (mcg)
0	Retinol (mcg)
27.25	BetaCaro (mcg)
0.21	Vit B1 (mg)
0.05	Vit B2 (mg)
0.73	Vit B3 (mg)
1.36	Vit B3-NE (mg)
0.12	Vit B6 (mg)
0	Vit B12 (mcg)
0.02	Biot (mcg)
3.76	Vit C (mg)
0	Vit D-IU (IU)
0	Vit D-mcg (mcg)

2.06	Vit E-a-Toco (mg)
113.32	Folate (mcg)
11.06	Vit K (mcg)
0.31	Panto (mg)
26.4	Calc (mg)
0	Chrom (mcg)
0.25	Copp (mg)
0.01	Fluor (mg)
6.25	Iodine (mcg)
1.4	Iron (mg)
22.62	Magn (mg)
4.01	Mang (mg)
0	Moly (mcg)
108.37	Phos (mg)
186.66	Pot (mg)
2.7	Sel (mcg)
32.08	Sod (mg)
0.88	Zinc (mg)
0.58	Omega3 (g)
3.86	Omega6 (g)
19.19	Chln (mg)

Citrus Guacamole

Total	Item Name Citrus Guacamole
1	Quantity
Serving = 2 tbsp	Measure
57.69	Cals (kcal)
0.81	Prot (g)
3.8	Carb (g)
2.44	TotFib (g)
0.62	Sugar (g)
0	SugAdd (g)
4.96	Fat (g)
0.72	SatFat (g)
3.29	MonoFat (g)
0.62	PolyFat (g)
0	TransFat (g)
0	Chol (mg)
259.95	Vit A-IU (IU)
13	Vit A-RAE (mcg)
25.99	Caroten (mcg)
0	Retinol (mcg)
131.97	BetaCaro (mcg)
0.03	Vit B1 (mg)
0.05	Vit B2 (mg)
0.67	Vit B3 (mg)
0.83	Vit B3-NE (mg)
0.11	Vit B6 (mg)
0	Vit B12 (mcg)
1.41	Biot (mcg)
11.61	Vit C (mg)
0	Vit D-IU (IU)
0	Vit D-mcg (mcg)
0.81	Vit E-a-Toco (mg)

30.66	Folate (mcg)
8.23	Vit K (mcg)
0.49	Panto (mg)
6.81	Calc (mg)
0.04	Chrom (mcg)
0.07	Copp (mg)
0.01	Fluor (mg)
4.89	Iodine (mcg)
0.28	Iron (mg)
11.28	Magn (mg)
0.06	Mang (mg)
0.5	Moly (mcg)
20.92	Phos (mg)
192.84	Pot (mg)
0.18	Sel (mcg)
19.05	Sod (mg)
0.24	Zinc (mg)
0.04	Omega3 (g)
0.57	Omega6 (g)
5.64	Chln (mg)

Heirloom Tomato & Avocado Bruschetta

Total	Item Name Heirloom Tomato & Avocado Bruschetta
1	Quantity
Serving	Measure
419.25	Cals (kcal)
15.4	Prot (g)
74.58	Carb (g)
4.13	TotFib (g)
7.2	Sugar (g)
0	SugAdd (g)
6.94	Fat (g)
1.14	SatFat (g)
2.45	MonoFat (g)
1.56	PolyFat (g)
0.01	TransFat (g)
0	Chol (mg)
315.58	Vit A-IU (IU)
15.78	Vit A-RAE (mcg)
31.56	Caroten (mcg)
0	Retinol (mcg)
167.58	BetaCaro (mcg)
1	Vit B1 (mg)
0.61	Vit B2 (mg)
7.02	Vit B3 (mg)
7.09	Vit B3-NE (mg)
0.21	Vit B6 (mg)
0	Vit B12 (mcg)
2.57	Biot (mcg)
8.57	Vit C (mg)
0	Vit D-IU (IU)
0	Vit D-mcg (mcg)
0.68	Vit E-a-Toco (mg)
184.39	Folate (mcg)
6.63	Vit K (mcg)
0.8	Panto (mg)
80.59	Calc (mg)
0.12	Chrom (mcg)
0.25	Copp (mg)
0.01	Fluor (mg)
14.49	Iodine (mcg)
5.69	Iron (mg)
50.28	Magn (mg)
0.85	Mang (mg)
1.2	Moly (mcg)
157.57	Phos (mg)
264.8	Pot (mg)
39.87	Sel (mcg)
926.27	Sod (mg)
1.56	Zinc (mg)
0.11	Omega3 (g)
1.29	Omega6 (g)
14.37	Chln (mg)

Nachos by Nature

Total	Item Name Nachos by Nature
1	Quantity
Serving	Measure
372.68	Cals (kcal)
8.37	Prot (g)
47.38	Carb (g)
8.88	TotFib (g)
4.76	Sugar (g)
0.57	SugAdd (g)
17.08	Fat (g)
3.24	SatFat (g)
5.73	MonoFat (g)
3.31	PolyFat (g)
0.02	TransFat (g)
0	Chol (mg)
926.28	Vit A-IU (IU)
46.31	Vit A-RAE (mcg)
92.63	Caroten (mcg)
0	Retinol (mcg)
378.03	BetaCaro (mcg)
0.22	Vit B1 (mg)
0.12	Vit B2 (mg)
1.87	Vit B3 (mg)
2.85	Vit B3-NE (mg)
0.26	Vit B6 (mg)
0	Vit B12 (mcg)
1.82	Biot (mcg)
23.29	Vit C (mg)
0.13	Vit D-IU (IU)
0	Vit D-mcg (mcg)
1.65	Vit E-a-Toco (mg)
107.91	Folate (mcg)
21.7	Vit K (mcg)
0.78	Panto (mg)
102.5	Calc (mg)
0.14	Chrom (mcg)
0.27	Copp (mg)
0.01	Fluor (mg)
3.53	Iodine (mcg)
2.18	Iron (mg)
68.26	Magn (mg)
0.54	Mang (mg)
1.79	Moly (mcg)
168.71	Phos (mg)
695.3	Pot (mg)
5.17	Sel (mcg)
322.6	Sod (mg)
1.31	Zinc (mg)
0.19	Omega3 (g)
3.12	Omega6 (g)
23.98	Chln (mg)

Please Note, nutritional vaules of all recipes may vary depending on the type of ingredients used "Nutritional analysis from Food Processor® Nutrition and Fitness Software version 11.5, ©2018 ESHA Research, Inc."

Peaceful Plates

Coconut Chickpea & Vegetable Curry with Quinoa

Total	Item Name Coconut Chickpea & Vegetable Curry with Quinoa
1	Quantity
Serving	Measure
415.59	Cals (kcal)
13.2	Prot (g)
50.8	Carb (g)
9.25	TotFib (g)
1.46	TotSolFib (g)
7.94	Sugar (g)
0	SugAdd (g)
19.74	Fat (g)
14.4	SatFat (g)
1.54	MonoFat (g)
1.88	PolyFat (g)
0	TransFat (g)
0	Chol (mg)
8441.34	Vit A-IU (IU)
422.07	Vit A-RAE (mcg)
844.13	Caroten (mcg)
0	Retinol (mcg)
3847.79	BetaCaro (mcg)
0.34	Vit B1 (mg)
0.28	Vit B2 (mg)
2.73	Vit B3 (mg)
5.07	Vit B3-NE (mg)
0.51	Vit B6 (mg)
0.01	Vit B12 (mcg)
0.87	Biot (mcg)

Total	Item Name
51.19	Vit C (mg)
0.4	Vit D-IU (IU)
0.01	Vit D-mcg (mcg)
1.98	Vit E-a-Toco (mg)
246.84	Folate (mcg)
38.28	Vit K (mcg)
1.37	Panto (mg)
105.99	Calc (mg)
0.12	Chrom (mcg)
0.61	Copp (mg)
0.01	Fluor (mg)
9.39	Iodine (mcg)
6	Iron (mg)
131.36	Magn (mg)
6.64	Mang (mg)
6.21	Moly (mcg)
320.47	Phos (mg)
949.32	Pot (mg)
7.08	Sel (mcg)
425.11	Sod (mg)
2.38	Zinc (mg)
0.13	Omega3 (g)
1.75	Omega6 (g)
63.22	Chln (mg)

Not so Dull, Dhal

Total	Item Name Not so Dull, Dhal
1	Quantity
Serving	Measure
396.25	Cals (kcal)
15.08	Prot (g)
66.59	Carb (g)
10.01	TotFib (g)
0	TotSolFib (g)
4.75	Sugar (g)
0	SugAdd (g)
8.1	Fat (g)
6	SatFat (g)
0.33	MonoFat (g)
0.09	PolyFat (g)
0	TransFat (g)
0	Chol (mg)
428.51	Vit A-IU (IU)
21.43	Vit A-RAE (mcg)
42.85	Caroten (mcg)
0	Retinol (mcg)
0.26	BetaCaro (mcg)
0.08	Vit B1 (mg)
0.01	Vit B2 (mg)
0.19	Vit B3 (mg)
0.34	Vit B3-NE (mg)
0.05	Vit B6 (mg)
0	Vit B12 (mcg)
0.7	Biot (mcg)
14.41	Vit C (mg)
0	Vit D-IU (IU)
0	Vit D-mcg (mcg)

0.01	Vit E-a-Toco (mg)
7.26	Folate (mcg)
0.11	Vit K (mcg)
0.07	Panto (mg)
76.05	Calc (mg)
0	Chrom (mcg)
0.07	Copp (mg)
0.01	Fluor (mg)
6.65	Iodine (mcg)
4.17	Iron (mg)
13.6	Magn (mg)
0.23	Mang (mg)
1	Moly (mcg)
30.7	Phos (mg)
698.77	Pot (mg)
0.27	Sel (mcg)
301.68	Sod (mg)
0.18	Zinc (mg)
0	Omega3 (g)
0.09	Omega6 (g)
3.73	Chln (mg)

Miso & Orange Crispy Asian Tofu Stir Fry

Total	Item Name Miso & Orange Crispy Asian Tofu Stir Fry
1	Quantity
Serving	Measure
513.01	Cals (kcal)
20.49	Prot (g)
61.03	Carb (g)
7.97	TotFib (g)
0.87	TotSolFib (g)
13.11	Sugar (g)
5.99	SugAdd (g)
21.83	Fat (g)
3.34	SatFat (g)
8.72	MonoFat (g)
6.42	PolyFat (g)
0	TransFat (g)
0	Chol (mg)
6194.03	Vit A-IU (IU)
309.83	Vit A-RAE (mcg)
619.4	Caroten (mcg)
0	Retinol (mcg)
3076.78	BetaCaro (mcg)
0.43	Vit B1 (mg)
0.4	Vit B2 (mg)
5.34	Vit B3 (mg)
7.87	Vit B3-NE (mg)
0.55	Vit B6 (mg)
0.01	Vit B12 (mcg)
2.01	Biot (mcg)
51.25	Vit C (mg)
0.27	Vit D-IU (IU)
0.01	Vit D-mcg (mcg)
1.11	Vit E-a-Toco (mg)
148.39	Folate (mcg)
22.82	Vit K (mcg)
1.14	Panto (mg)
151.55	Calc (mg)
0.35	Chrom (mcg)
0.44	Copp (mg)
0.01	Fluor (mg)
7.31	Iodine (mcg)
4.05	Iron (mg)
116.5	Magn (mg)
2.27	Mang (mg)
6.28	Moly (mcg)
303.62	Phos (mg)
687.84	Pot (mg)
13.04	Sel (mcg)
1260.21	Sod (mg)
2.33	Zinc (mg)
0.14	Omega3 (g)
2.69	Omega6 (g)
49.68	Chln (mg)

Cool Beans Chili

Total	Item Name Cool Beans Chili
1	Quantity
Serving = 1 cup	Measure
251.08	Cals (kcal)
10.33	Prot (g)
41.71	Carb (g)
9.94	TotFib (g)
1.21	TotSolFib (g)
7.72	Sugar (g)
1.13	SugAdd (g)
5.45	Fat (g)
0.88	SatFat (g)
1.8	MonoFat (g)
0.64	PolyFat (g)
0	TransFat (g)
0	Chol (mg)
1436.15	Vit A-IU (IU)
71.81	Vit A-RAE (mcg)
143.61	Caroten (mcg)
0	Retinol (mcg)
565.39	BetaCaro (mcg)
0.32	Vit B1 (mg)
0.15	Vit B2 (mg)
1.85	Vit B3 (mg)
3.58	Vit B3-NE (mg)
0.25	Vit B6 (mg)
0.01	Vit B12 (mcg)
0.6	Biot (mcg)
37.34	Vit C (mg)
0.25	Vit D-IU (IU)
0.01	Vit D-mcg (mcg)

0.46	Vit E-a-Toco (mg)
158.4	Folate (mcg)
30.09	Vit K (mcg)
0.6	Panto (mg)
108.7	Calc (mg)
0.07	Chrom (mcg)
0.36	Copp (mg)
0.01	Fluor (mg)
6.05	Iodine (mcg)
2.74	Iron (mg)
72.37	Magn (mg)
0.78	Mang (mg)
2.04	Moly (mcg)
175.2	Phos (mg)
960.71	Pot (mg)
5.51	Sel (mcg)
94.65	Sod (mg)
1.45	Zinc (mg)
0.14	Omega3 (g)
0.51	Omega6 (g)
28.27	Chln (mg)

Timeless Tacos

Total	Item Name Timeless Tacos
1	Quantity
Serving = 1 taco	Measure
276.21	Cals (kcal)
7.87	Prot (g)
36.96	Carb (g)
8.29	TotFib (g)
0.4	TotSolFib (g)
5.27	Sugar (g)
0.38	SugAdd (g)
11.77	Fat (g)
2.37	SatFat (g)
5.53	MonoFat (g)
1.15	PolyFat (g)
0	TransFat (g)
0	Chol (mg)
887.33	Vit A-IU (IU)
44.37	Vit A-RAE (mcg)
88.73	Caroten (mcg)
0	Retinol (mcg)
398.3	BetaCaro (mcg)
0.16	Vit B1 (mg)
0.13	Vit B2 (mg)
1.68	Vit B3 (mg)
2.53	Vit B3-NE (mg)
0.26	Vit B6 (mg)
0	Vit B12 (mcg)
2.68	Biot (mcg)
28.77	Vit C (mg)
0.08	Vit D-IU (IU)
0	Vit D-mcg (mcg)

1.4	Vit E-a-Toco (mg)
101.81	Folate (mcg)
23.01	Vit K (mcg)
0.96	Panto (mg)
49.61	Calc (mg)
0.17	Chrom (mcg)
0.24	Copp (mg)
0.01	Fluor (mg)
7.17	Iodine (mcg)
1.35	Iron (mg)
43.25	Magn (mg)
0.38	Mang (mg)
2.6	Moly (mcg)
95.49	Phos (mg)
649.33	Pot (mg)
2.15	Sel (mcg)
343.05	Sod (mg)
0.88	Zinc (mg)
0.11	Omega3 (g)
1.03	Omega6 (g)
19.26	Chln (mg)

Roasted Corn Salsa

Total	Item Name Roasted Corn Salsa
1	Quantity
Serving = 2 tbsp	Measure
25.39	Cals (kcal)
0.53	Prot (g)
3.43	Carb (g)
0.52	TotFib (g)
0	TotSolFib (g)
0.77	Sugar (g)
0	SugAdd (g)
1.34	Fat (g)
0.16	SatFat (g)
0.87	MonoFat (g)
0.24	PolyFat (g)
0	TransFat (g)
0	Chol (mg)
134.75	Vit A-IU (IU)
6.74	Vit A-RAE (mcg)
13.48	Caroten (mcg)
0	Retinol (mcg)
70.77	BetaCaro (mcg)
0.03	Vit B1 (mg)
0.01	Vit B2 (mg)
0.27	Vit B3 (mg)
0.34	Vit B3-NE (mg)
0.03	Vit B6 (mg)
0	Vit B12 (mcg)
0.12	Biot (mcg)
6.98	Vit C (mg)
0	Vit D-IU (IU)
0	Vit D-mcg (mcg)

0.1	Vit E-a-Toco (mg)
8.59	Folate (mcg)
0.64	Vit K (mcg)
0.12	Panto (mg)
2.47	Calc (mg)
--	Chrom (mcg)
0.01	Copp (mg)
0	Fluor (mg)
0.1	Iodine (mcg)
0.11	Iron (mg)
6.08	Magn (mg)
0.04	Mang (mg)
0.32	Moly (mcg)
14.49	Phos (mg)
55.02	Pot (mg)
0.14	Sel (mcg)
2.41	Sod (mg)
0.08	Zinc (mg)
0.02	Omega3 (g)
0.22	Omega6 (g)
0.75	Chln (mg)

BBQ "you don't know" Jackfruit Sliders with Country Slaw

Total	Item Name BBQ "you don't know" Jackfruit Sliders with Country Slaw
1	Quantity
Serving	Measure
189.75	Cals (kcal)
3.45	Prot (g)
31.95	Carb (g)
2.15	TotFib (g)
0.71	TotSolFib (g)
19.75	Sugar (g)
2.58	SugAdd (g)
6.46	Fat (g)
0.9	SatFat (g)
3.95	MonoFat (g)
1.08	PolyFat (g)
0	TransFat (g)
0	Chol (mg)
547.42	Vit A-IU (IU)
31.28	Vit A-RAE (mcg)
52.98	Caroten (mcg)
4.79	Retinol (mcg)
284.88	BetaCaro (mcg)
0.18	Vit B1 (mg)
0.1	Vit B2 (mg)
1.42	Vit B3 (mg)
1.86	Vit B3-NE (mg)
0.28	Vit B6 (mg)
0.03	Vit B12 (mcg)
0.55	Biot (mcg)
15.46	Vit C (mg)

Total	Item Name
0	Vit D-IU (IU)
0	Vit D-mcg (mcg)
0.32	Vit E-a-Toco (mg)
36.59	Folate (mcg)
9.98	Vit K (mcg)
0.3	Panto (mg)
66.05	Calc (mg)
0.01	Chrom (mcg)
0.12	Copp (mg)
0.01	Fluor (mg)
8.22	Iodine (mcg)
1.28	Iron (mg)
30.49	Magn (mg)
0.19	Mang (mg)
0.7	Moly (mcg)
38	Phos (mg)
465.8	Pot (mg)
5.08	Sel (mcg)
142.92	Sod (mg)
0.27	Zinc (mg)
0.14	Omega3 (g)
0.94	Omega6 (g)
4.06	Chln (mg)

Pacific Coast Black Bean Burgers
with Pineapple Salsa

Total	Item Name Pacific Coast Black Bean Burgers with Pineapple Salsa
1	Quantity
Serving = 1 burger	Measure
478.09	Cals (kcal)
18.74	Prot (g)
79.88	Carb (g)
14.14	TotFib (g)
1.47	TotSolFib (g)
17.41	Sugar (g)
1.7	SugAdd (g)
11.22	Fat (g)
1.65	SatFat (g)
4.31	MonoFat (g)
3.88	PolyFat (g)
0.01	TransFat (g)
0	Chol (mg)
1670.21	Vit A-IU (IU)
93.92	Vit A-RAE (mcg)
162.31	Caroten (mcg)
12.76	Retinol (mcg)
909.89	BetaCaro (mcg)
0.89	Vit B1 (mg)
0.3	Vit B2 (mg)
3.82	Vit B3 (mg)
6.46	Vit B3-NE (mg)
0.44	Vit B6 (mg)
0.09	Vit B12 (mcg)
1.6	Biot (mcg)

76.05	Vit C (mg)
0	Vit D-IU (IU)
0	Vit D-mcg (mcg)
0.86	Vit E-a-Toco (mg)
302.58	Folate (mcg)
133.71	Vit K (mcg)
1.09	Panto (mg)
210.55	Calc (mg)
0	Chrom (mcg)
0.7	Copp (mg)
0.04	Fluor (mg)
43.58	Iodine (mcg)
6.66	Iron (mg)
153.41	Magn (mg)
1.78	Mang (mg)
2.07	Moly (mcg)
314.2	Phos (mg)
1241	Pot (mg)
16.38	Sel (mcg)
393.31	Sod (mg)
2.87	Zinc (mg)
1.84	Omega3 (g)
1.37	Omega6 (g)
53.78	Chln (mg)

Bean & Avocado Cashewdillas
with Peach Salsa

Total	Item Name Bean & Avocado Cashewdillas with Peach Salsa
1	Quantity
Serving = 1 Cashewdillas	Measure
632.81	Cals (kcal)
21.19	Prot (g)
93.33	Carb (g)
14.64	TotFib (g)
1.89	TotSolFib (g)
15.47	Sugar (g)
0	SugAdd (g)
22.97	Fat (g)
4.68	SatFat (g)
10.74	MonoFat (g)
2.97	PolyFat (g)
0	TransFat (g)
0	Chol (mg)
2328.8	Vit A-IU (IU)
116.44	Vit A-RAE (mcg)
232.88	Caroten (mcg)
0	Retinol (mcg)
1206.94	BetaCaro (mcg)
1.33	Vit B1 (mg)
1.07	Vit B2 (mg)
7.73	Vit B3 (mg)
10.65	Vit B3-NE (mg)
1.06	Vit B6 (mg)
1.33	Vit B12 (mcg)
5.97	Biot (mcg)
75.62	Vit C (mg)
0.54	Vit D-IU (IU)
0.02	Vit D-mcg (mcg)
3.14	Vit E-a-Toco (mg)
231.21	Folate (mcg)
29.05	Vit K (mcg)
1.9	Panto (mg)
78.62	Calc (mg)
0.32	Chrom (mcg)
0.85	Copp (mg)
0.07	Fluor (mg)
63.05	Iodine (mcg)
4.89	Iron (mg)
136.1	Magn (mg)
0.97	Mang (mg)
5.79	Moly (mcg)
349.99	Phos (mg)
1409.58	Pot (mg)
9.45	Sel (mcg)
900.81	Sod (mg)
2.94	Zinc (mg)
0.25	Omega3 (g)
2.71	Omega6 (g)
48.09	Chln (mg)

Oven Roasted Eggplant & Tomato Panini

Total	Item Name Panini
1	Quantity
Serving = 1 panini	Measure
915.07	Cals (kcal)
33.67	Prot (g)
158.76	Carb (g)
11.79	TotFib (g)
1.97	TotSolFib (g)
20.02	Sugar (g)
0	SugAdd (g)
17.89	Fat (g)
3.08	SatFat (g)
8.64	MonoFat (g)
4.11	PolyFat (g)
0.02	TransFat (g)
0	Chol (mg)
1662.14	Vit A-IU (IU)
83.11	Vit A-RAE (mcg)
166.21	Caroten (mcg)
0	Retinol (mcg)
949.99	BetaCaro (mcg)
3.56	Vit B1 (mg)
2.49	Vit B2 (mg)
20.73	Vit B3 (mg)
21.11	Vit B3-NE (mg)
1.28	Vit B6 (mg)
2.19	Vit B12 (mcg)
8.26	Biot (mcg)
30.21	Vit C (mg)
0	Vit D-IU (IU)
0	Vit D-mcg (mcg)
1.59	Vit E-a-Toco (mg)
408.12	Folate (mcg)
149.4	Vit K (mcg)
1.85	Panto (mg)
199.72	Calc (mg)
0.63	Chrom (mcg)
0.62	Copp (mg)
0.01	Fluor (mg)
27.57	Iodine (mcg)
12.22	Iron (mg)
130.44	Magn (mg)
2.14	Mang (mg)
11.35	Moly (mcg)
377.22	Phos (mg)
983.94	Pot (mg)
80.39	Sel (mcg)
1739.44	Sod (mg)
3.67	Zinc (mg)
0.22	Omega3 (g)
2.38	Omega6 (g)
41.23	Chln (mg)

Tahini & Lentil Falafel Wrap with Roasted Red Pepper Dressing

Total	Item Name Tahini & Lentil Falafel Wrap with Roasted Red Pepper Dressing
1	Quantity
Serving = 1 wrap	Measure
607.68	Cals (kcal)
25.38	Prot (g)
90.56	Carb (g)
12.14	TotFib (g)
1.23	TotSolFib (g)
11.36	Sugar (g)
0	SugAdd (g)
18.51	Fat (g)
3.89	SatFat (g)
5.47	MonoFat (g)
4.91	PolyFat (g)
0	TransFat (g)
0	Chol (mg)
8245.26	Vit A-IU (IU)
412.28	Vit A-RAE (mcg)
824.56	Caroten (mcg)
0	Retinol (mcg)
4256.11	BetaCaro (mcg)
0.57	Vit B1 (mg)
0.23	Vit B2 (mg)
3.11	Vit B3 (mg)
6.09	Vit B3-NE (mg)
0.68	Vit B6 (mg)
0	Vit B12 (mcg)
2.63	Biot (mcg)
112.55	Vit C (mg)
0	Vit D-IU (IU)
0	Vit D-mcg (mcg)
2.39	Vit E-a-Toco (mg)
272.93	Folate (mcg)
166.29	Vit K (mcg)
1.04	Panto (mg)
112.86	Calc (mg)
0.43	Chrom (mcg)
1.04	Copp (mg)
0.02	Fluor (mg)
20.94	Iodine (mcg)
6.85	Iron (mg)
124.84	Magn (mg)
5.73	Mang (mg)
8.9	Moly (mcg)
382.01	Phos (mg)
1052.82	Pot (mg)
4.18	Sel (mcg)
751.74	Sod (mg)
3.59	Zinc (mg)
0.63	Omega3 (g)
4.28	Omega6 (g)
35.74	Chln (mg)

Sprouted Spelt Flour Pizza

Total	Item Name Sprouted Spelt Flour Pizza
1	Quantity
Serving = 1 slice	Measure
287.12	Cals (kcal)
6.69	Prot (g)
35.8	Carb (g)
7.5	TotFib (g)
0.02	TotSolFib (g)
5.62	Sugar (g)
1.14	SugAdd (g)
12.87	Fat (g)
2.41	SatFat (g)
5.05	MonoFat (g)
1.58	PolyFat (g)
0	TransFat (g)
0	Chol (mg)
1317.55	Vit A-IU (IU)
65.88	Vit A-RAE (mcg)
131.76	Caroten (mcg)
0	Retinol (mcg)
690.1	BetaCaro (mcg)
0.17	Vit B1 (mg)
0.12	Vit B2 (mg)
1.22	Vit B3 (mg)
1.65	Vit B3-NE (mg)
0.14	Vit B6 (mg)
0.01	Vit B12 (mcg)
1.38	Biot (mcg)
39.98	Vit C (mg)
0.25	Vit D-IU (IU)

0.01	Vit D-mcg (mcg)
0.96	Vit E-a-Toco (mg)
51.51	Folate (mcg)
41.48	Vit K (mcg)
0.37	Panto (mg)
61.86	Calc (mg)
0.12	Chrom (mcg)
0.15	Copp (mg)
0.04	Fluor (mg)
35.08	Iodine (mcg)
2.36	Iron (mg)
26.64	Magn (mg)
0.35	Mang (mg)
2.86	Moly (mcg)
51.74	Phos (mg)
345.4	Pot (mg)
3.38	Sel (mcg)
513.96	Sod (mg)
0.43	Zinc (mg)
0.56	Omega3 (g)
0.31	Omega6 (g)
11.96	Chln (mg)

Pronoto Pasta Primavera

Total	Item Name **Pronoto Pasta Primavera**
1	Quantity
Serving	Measure
381.03	Cals (kcal)
13.63	Prot (g)
70.58	Carb (g)
6.8	TotFib (g)
1.17	TotSolFib (g)
9.24	Sugar (g)
0	SugAdd (g)
4.86	Fat (g)
0.76	SatFat (g)
2.58	MonoFat (g)
0.99	PolyFat (g)
0	TransFat (g)
0	Chol (mg)
2414.17	Vit A-IU (IU)
120.71	Vit A-RAE (mcg)
241.42	Caroten (mcg)
0	Retinol (mcg)
1157.34	BetaCaro (mcg)
2.05	Vit B1 (mg)
1.54	Vit B2 (mg)
11.86	Vit B3 (mg)
14.53	Vit B3-NE (mg)
0.98	Vit B6 (mg)
1.96	Vit B12 (mcg)
3.55	Biot (mcg)
57.41	Vit C (mg)
0.4	Vit D-IU (IU)
0.01	Vit D-mcg (mcg)

1.27	Vit E-a-Toco (mg)
227.59	Folate (mcg)
58.8	Vit K (mcg)
0.75	Panto (mg)
91.16	Calc (mg)
0.03	Chrom (mcg)
0.37	Copp (mg)
0.02	Fluor (mg)
4.52	Iodine (mcg)
3.63	Iron (mg)
67.5	Magn (mg)
0.97	Mang (mg)
6	Moly (mcg)
212.37	Phos (mg)
839.8	Pot (mg)
51.91	Sel (mcg)
63.47	Sod (mg)
1.74	Zinc (mg)
0.06	Omega3 (g)
0.46	Omega6 (g)
26.6	Chln (mg)

Return of the Mac 'n' Cheese

Total	Item Name Return of the Mac 'n' Cheese
1	Quantity
Serving	Measure
230.11	Cals (kcal)
6.4	Prot (g)
16.53	Carb (g)
2.35	TotFib (g)
0	TotSolFib (g)
2.1	Sugar (g)
0	SugAdd (g)
16.73	Fat (g)
7.53	SatFat (g)
5.46	MonoFat (g)
2.35	PolyFat (g)
0	TransFat (g)
0	Chol (mg)
150.66	Vit A-IU (IU)
1.28	Vit A-RAE (mcg)
2.57	Caroten (mcg)
0	Retinol (mcg)
15.32	BetaCaro (mcg)
2.31	Vit B1 (mg)
1.97	Vit B2 (mg)
9.04	Vit B3 (mg)
9.92	Vit B3-NE (mg)
1.24	Vit B6 (mg)
4.04	Vit B12 (mcg)
3.29	Biot (mcg)
9.31	Vit C (mg)
25	Vit D-IU (IU)
0.62	Vit D-mcg (mcg)
1.86	Vit E-a-Toco (mg)
12.39	Folate (mcg)
5.67	Vit K (mcg)
0.26	Panto (mg)
139.96	Calc (mg)
0	Chrom (mcg)
0.44	Copp (mg)
0.01	Fluor (mg)
12.9	Iodine (mcg)
2.66	Iron (mg)
71.65	Magn (mg)
0.58	Mang (mg)
1	Moly (mcg)
158.3	Phos (mg)
425.94	Pot (mg)
3.71	Sel (mcg)
129.83	Sod (mg)
1.83	Zinc (mg)
0.01	Omega3 (g)
1.34	Omega6 (g)
4.31	Chln (mg)

Oven Roasted Tomato & Mushroom Alfredo

Total	Item Name Oven Roasted Tomato & Mushroom Alfredo
1	Quantity
Serving	Measure
486.12	Cals (kcal)
14.47	Prot (g)
72.29	Carb (g)
5.68	TotFib (g)
1.48	TotSolFib (g)
6.67	Sugar (g)
0	SugAdd (g)
14.35	Fat (g)
2.07	SatFat (g)
8.96	MonoFat (g)
2.19	PolyFat (g)
0.01	TransFat (g)
0	Chol (mg)
641.22	Vit A-IU (IU)
55.58	Vit A-RAE (mcg)
54.82	Caroten (mcg)
28.16	Retinol (mcg)
298.23	BetaCaro (mcg)
1.83	Vit B1 (mg)
1.36	Vit B2 (mg)
11.44	Vit B3 (mg)
14.52	Vit B3-NE (mg)
0.83	Vit B6 (mg)
1.5	Vit B12 (mcg)
4.96	Biot (mcg)
15.72	Vit C (mg)
28.59	Vit D-IU (IU)

0.69	Vit D-mcg (mcg)
3.95	Vit E-a-Toco (mg)
219.98	Folate (mcg)
21.71	Vit K (mcg)
1.23	Panto (mg)
180.73	Calc (mg)
0.42	Chrom (mcg)
0.67	Copp (mg)
0.02	Fluor (mg)
8.7	Iodine (mcg)
3.94	Iron (mg)
89.82	Magn (mg)
1.19	Mang (mg)
5.03	Moly (mcg)
294.42	Phos (mg)
770.3	Pot (mg)
59.22	Sel (mcg)
97.15	Sod (mg)
2.42	Zinc (mg)
0.1	Omega3 (g)
2.09	Omega6 (g)
26.81	Chln (mg)

Moroccan Sweet Potato & Black Bean Tagine

Total	Item Name Moroccan Sweet Potato & Black Bean Tagine
1	Quantity
Serving	Measure
584.43	Cals (kcal)
25.02	Prot (g)
112.62	Carb (g)
22.54	TotFib (g)
4.28	TotSolFib (g)
21.06	Sugar (g)
0	SugAdd (g)
6.05	Fat (g)
0.92	SatFat (g)
2.6	MonoFat (g)
1.46	PolyFat (g)
0	TransFat (g)
0	Chol (mg)
6992.06	Vit A-IU (IU)
349.6	Vit A-RAE (mcg)
699.21	Caroten (mcg)
0	Retinol (mcg)
4154.92	BetaCaro (mcg)
0.76	Vit B1 (mg)
0.31	Vit B2 (mg)
3.42	Vit B3 (mg)
8.09	Vit B3-NE (mg)
0.68	Vit B6 (mg)
0	Vit B12 (mcg)
3.4	Biot (mcg)
12.09	Vit C (mg)
0	Vit D-IU (IU)

0	Vit D-mcg (mcg)
1.42	Vit E-a-Toco (mg)
404.81	Folate (mcg)
27.01	Vit K (mcg)
1.72	Panto (mg)
201.75	Calc (mg)
0.34	Chrom (mcg)
0.92	Copp (mg)
0.07	Fluor (mg)
67.05	Iodine (mcg)
7.98	Iron (mg)
184.49	Magn (mg)
5.5	Mang (mg)
6.31	Moly (mcg)
451.7	Phos (mg)
1844.88	Pot (mg)
7.35	Sel (mcg)
316.96	Sod (mg)
3.43	Zinc (mg)
0.23	Omega3 (g)
1.23	Omega6 (g)
54.14	Chln (mg)

Please Note, nutritional vaules of all recipes may vary depending on the type of ingredients used "Nutritional analysis from Food Processor® Nutrition and Fitness Software version 11.5, ©2018 ESHA Research, Inc."

Sweet Street

Nanny's Oatmeal Chocolate Chip Cookies

Total	Item Name Nanny's Oatmeal Chocolate Chip Cookies
1	Quantity
Serving = 1 cookie	Measure
202.45	Cals (kcal)
2.82	Prot (g)
25.98	Carb (g)
2.43	TotFib (g)
13.57	Sugar (g)
8.77	SugAdd (g)
9.84	Fat (g)
3.92	SatFat (g)
1.77	MonoFat (g)
1.83	PolyFat (g)
0	TransFat (g)
0	Chol (mg)
0.32	Vit A-IU (IU)
0.02	Vit A-RAE (mcg)
0.03	Caroten (mcg)
0	Retinol (mcg)
0.12	BetaCaro (mcg)
0	Vit B1 (mg)
0	Vit B2 (mg)
0.01	Vit B3 (mg)
0.03	Vit B3-NE (mg)
0	Vit B6 (mg)
0	Vit B12 (mcg)
--	Biot (mcg)
0.01	Vit C (mg)
0	Vit D-IU (IU)

0	Vit D-mcg (mcg)
0	Vit E-a-Toco (mg)
0.26	Folate (mcg)
0.05	Vit K (mcg)
0	Panto (mg)
30.77	Calc (mg)
--	Chrom (mcg)
0	Copp (mg)
--	Fluor (mg)
--	Iodine (mcg)
1.68	Iron (mg)
16.06	Magn (mg)
0.03	Mang (mg)
--	Moly (mcg)
45.43	Phos (mg)
43.38	Pot (mg)
0.08	Sel (mcg)
104.3	Sod (mg)
0.44	Zinc (mg)
0.07	Omega3 (g)
0.02	Omega6 (g)
0.24	Chln (mg)

High Vibing Bean & Molasses Cookies

Total	Item Name High Vibing Bean & Molasses Cookies
1	Quantity
Serving = 1 cookie	Measure
193.79	Cals (kcal)
4.56	Prot (g)
21.51	Carb (g)
3.42	TotFib (g)
8.38	Sugar (g)
4.2	SugAdd (g)
10.53	Fat (g)
6.03	SatFat (g)
1.29	MonoFat (g)
1.45	PolyFat (g)
0	TransFat (g)
0	Chol (mg)
3.91	Vit A-IU (IU)
0.2	Vit A-RAE (mcg)
0.39	Caroten (mcg)
0	Retinol (mcg)
1.36	BetaCaro (mcg)
0.12	Vit B1 (mg)
0.03	Vit B2 (mg)
0.56	Vit B3 (mg)
1.24	Vit B3-NE (mg)
0.09	Vit B6 (mg)
0	Vit B12 (mcg)
--	Biot (mcg)
0.14	Vit C (mg)
0	Vit D-IU (IU)
0	Vit D-mcg (mcg)

1.21	Vit E-a-Toco (mg)
37.94	Folate (mcg)
0.62	Vit K (mcg)
0.16	Panto (mg)
47.89	Calc (mg)
0	Chrom (mcg)
0.22	Copp (mg)
0	Fluor (mg)
1.75	Iodine (mcg)
2.14	Iron (mg)
51.91	Magn (mg)
0.42	Mang (mg)
0	Moly (mcg)
97.55	Phos (mg)
287.91	Pot (mg)
3.21	Sel (mcg)
55.05	Sod (mg)
0.85	Zinc (mg)
0.13	Omega3 (g)
1.32	Omega6 (g)
8.4	Chln (mg)

No Frownies with these Brownies

Total	Item Name No Frownies with these Brownies
1	Quantity
Serving	Measure
185.98	Cals (kcal)
2.57	Prot (g)
16.13	Carb (g)
1.64	TotFib (g)
10.95	Sugar (g)
9.69	SugAdd (g)
13	Fat (g)
6.11	SatFat (g)
0.79	MonoFat (g)
1.97	PolyFat (g)
0	TransFat (g)
0	Chol (mg)
5.45	Vit A-IU (IU)
0.27	Vit A-RAE (mcg)
0.55	Caroten (mcg)
0	Retinol (mcg)
2.36	BetaCaro (mcg)
0.02	Vit B1 (mg)
0.01	Vit B2 (mg)
0.1	Vit B3 (mg)
0.24	Vit B3-NE (mg)
0.05	Vit B6 (mg)
0	Vit B12 (mcg)
0.89	Biot (mcg)
0.69	Vit C (mg)
0	Vit D-IU (IU)
0	Vit D-mcg (mcg)

0.04	Vit E-a-Toco (mg)
5.44	Folate (mcg)
0.2	Vit K (mcg)
0.05	Panto (mg)
36.69	Calc (mg)
0.06	Chrom (mcg)
0.07	Copp (mg)
0	Fluor (mg)
4.04	Iodine (mcg)
1.3	Iron (mg)
9.52	Magn (mg)
0.16	Mang (mg)
1.08	Moly (mcg)
17.1	Phos (mg)
46.58	Pot (mg)
0.36	Sel (mcg)
61.05	Sod (mg)
0.14	Zinc (mg)
0.44	Omega3 (g)
1.54	Omega6 (g)
2.52	Chln (mg)

Double Chocolate Cake with Chocolate Avocado Icing

Total	Item Name Double Chocolate Cake with Chocolate Avocado Icing
1	Quantity
Serving	Measure
349.78	Cals (kcal)
4.48	Prot (g)
43.33	Carb (g)
5.48	TotFib (g)
22.95	Sugar (g)
22.87	SugAdd (g)
17.2	Fat (g)
10.49	SatFat (g)
3.19	MonoFat (g)
0.84	PolyFat (g)
0	TransFat (g)
0	Chol (mg)
64.32	Vit A-IU (IU)
11.05	Vit A-RAE (mcg)
3.33	Caroten (mcg)
9.39	Retinol (mcg)
14.28	BetaCaro (mcg)
0.04	Vit B1 (mg)
0.06	Vit B2 (mg)
0.51	Vit B3 (mg)
0.63	Vit B3-NE (mg)
0.07	Vit B6 (mg)
0	Vit B12 (mcg)
0.82	Biot (mcg)
2	Vit C (mg)
9.17	Vit D-IU (IU)

0.22	Vit D-mcg (mcg)
1.08	Vit E-a-Toco (mg)
21.29	Folate (mcg)
4.88	Vit K (mcg)
0.39	Panto (mg)
50.59	Calc (mg)
0	Chrom (mcg)
0.06	Copp (mg)
0.02	Fluor (mg)
4.62	Iodine (mcg)
3.29	Iron (mg)
11.54	Magn (mg)
0.08	Mang (mg)
0	Moly (mcg)
19.11	Phos (mg)
151.99	Pot (mg)
0.31	Sel (mcg)
349.93	Sod (mg)
0.21	Zinc (mg)
0.16	Omega3 (g)
0.67	Omega6 (g)
4.23	Chln (mg)

In a Pinch Blueberry Crisp

Total	Item Name In a Pinch Blueberry Crisp
1	Quantity
Serving	Measure
251.86	Cals (kcal)
2.39	Prot (g)
34.85	Carb (g)
4.52	TotFib (g)
21.15	Sugar (g)
10.89	SugAdd (g)
12.42	Fat (g)
9.62	SatFat (g)
0.71	MonoFat (g)
0.32	PolyFat (g)
0	TransFat (g)
0	Chol (mg)
54.71	Vit A-IU (IU)
2.74	Vit A-RAE (mcg)
5.47	Caroten (mcg)
0	Retinol (mcg)
32.08	BetaCaro (mcg)
0.04	Vit B1 (mg)
0.04	Vit B2 (mg)
0.44	Vit B3 (mg)
0.53	Vit B3-NE (mg)
0.06	Vit B6 (mg)
0	Vit B12 (mcg)
0.01	Biot (mcg)
10.62	Vit C (mg)
0	Vit D-IU (IU)
0	Vit D-mcg (mcg)
0.6	Vit E-a-Toco (mg)
6.75	Folate (mcg)
19.24	Vit K (mcg)
0.15	Panto (mg)
33.46	Calc (mg)
0	Chrom (mcg)
0.08	Copp (mg)
0	Fluor (mg)
4.27	Iodine (mcg)
1.15	Iron (mg)
25.3	Magn (mg)
0.5	Mang (mg)
0	Moly (mcg)
64.43	Phos (mg)
141.66	Pot (mg)
0.73	Sel (mcg)
26.08	Sod (mg)
0.5	Zinc (mg)
0.06	Omega3 (g)
0.26	Omega6 (g)
6.86	Chln (mg)

Chocolate Orange Avocado Pudding

Total	Item Name Chocolate Orange Avocado Pudding
1	Quantity
Serving	Measure
238.02	Cals (kcal)
3.2	Prot (g)
26.41	Carb (g)
7.54	TotFib (g)
13.12	Sugar (g)
11.98	SugAdd (g)
14.71	Fat (g)
1.93	SatFat (g)
8.92	MonoFat (g)
1.66	PolyFat (g)
0	TransFat (g)
0	Chol (mg)
164.36	Vit A-IU (IU)
7.7	Vit A-RAE (mcg)
15.39	Caroten (mcg)
0	Retinol (mcg)
60.53	BetaCaro (mcg)
0.09	Vit B1 (mg)
0.4	Vit B2 (mg)
1.79	Vit B3 (mg)
2.17	Vit B3-NE (mg)
0.26	Vit B6 (mg)
0.06	Vit B12 (mcg)
3.32	Biot (mcg)
13.15	Vit C (mg)
2.08	Vit D-IU (IU)
0.05	Vit D-mcg (mcg)
1.93	Vit E-a-Toco (mg)
83.79	Folate (mcg)
19.05	Vit K (mcg)
1.35	Panto (mg)
44.77	Calc (mg)
0.09	Chrom (mcg)
0.16	Copp (mg)
0.02	Fluor (mg)
18.69	Iodine (mcg)
3	Iron (mg)
31.99	Magn (mg)
0.6	Mang (mg)
0	Moly (mcg)
50.72	Phos (mg)
526.66	Pot (mg)
0.37	Sel (mcg)
76.26	Sod (mg)
0.79	Zinc (mg)
0.11	Omega3 (g)
1.52	Omega6 (g)
13.52	Chln (mg)

Coconut & Chocolate Mousse

Total	Item Name Coconut & Chocolate Mousse
1	Quantity
Serving	Measure
333.47	Cals (kcal)
4.87	Prot (g)
30.23	Carb (g)
7.54	TotFib (g)
15.98	Sugar (g)
15.98	SugAdd (g)
23.66	Fat (g)
13.83	SatFat (g)
0.66	MonoFat (g)
0.98	PolyFat (g)
0	TransFat (g)
0	Chol (mg)
1.89	Vit A-IU (IU)
0.09	Vit A-RAE (mcg)
0.19	Caroten (mcg)
0	Retinol (mcg)
0	BetaCaro (mcg)
0.05	Vit B1 (mg)
0.34	Vit B2 (mg)
0.74	Vit B3 (mg)
1.19	Vit B3-NE (mg)
0.02	Vit B6 (mg)
0	Vit B12 (mcg)
--	Biot (mcg)
4.69	Vit C (mg)
0	Vit D-IU (IU)
0	Vit D-mcg (mcg)

0.02	Vit E-a-Toco (mg)
10.63	Folate (mcg)
--	Vit K (mcg)
0.1	Panto (mg)
62.61	Calc (mg)
--	Chrom (mcg)
0.17	Copp (mg)
--	Fluor (mg)
--	Iodine (mcg)
4.8	Iron (mg)
46.62	Magn (mg)
1.2	Mang (mg)
--	Moly (mcg)
91.24	Phos (mg)
214.35	Pot (mg)
1.93	Sel (mcg)
11.24	Sod (mg)
0.7	Zinc (mg)
0.62	Omega3 (g)
0.35	Omega6 (g)
5.41	Chln (mg)

Strawberry Yogurt Popsicles

Total	Item Name Strawberry Yogurt Popsicles
1	Quantity
Serving = 1 popsicle	Measure
35.85	Cals (kcal)
1.74	Prot (g)
5.54	Carb (g)
0.92	TotFib (g)
2.39	Sugar (g)
0	SugAdd (g)
0.86	Fat (g)
0.11	SatFat (g)
0.23	MonoFat (g)
0.46	PolyFat (g)
0	TransFat (g)
0	Chol (mg)
17.66	Vit A-IU (IU)
4.8	Vit A-RAE (mcg)
0.22	Caroten (mcg)
4.69	Retinol (mcg)
1.26	BetaCaro (mcg)
0.04	Vit B1 (mg)
0.01	Vit B2 (mg)
0.18	Vit B3 (mg)
0.43	Vit B3-NE (mg)
0.02	Vit B6 (mg)
0.01	Vit B12 (mcg)
0.2	Biot (mcg)
29.41	Vit C (mg)
4.58	Vit D-IU (IU)
0.11	Vit D-mcg (mcg)
4.43	Vit E-a-Toco (mg)
8.19	Folate (mcg)
1.86	Vit K (mcg)
0.03	Panto (mg)
52.42	Calc (mg)
--	Chrom (mcg)
0.07	Copp (mg)
0	Fluor (mg)
1.62	Iodine (mcg)
0.45	Iron (mg)
13.56	Magn (mg)
0.25	Mang (mg)
--	Moly (mcg)
33.86	Phos (mg)
108.5	Pot (mg)
0.72	Sel (mcg)
11.28	Sod (mg)
0.23	Zinc (mg)
0.06	Omega3 (g)
0.4	Omega6 (g)
1.03	Chln (mg)

Blueberry Yogurt Popsicles

Total	Item Name Blueberry Yogurt Popsicles
1	Quantity
Serving = 1 popsicle	Measure
40.64	Cals (kcal)
1.76	Prot (g)
6.84	Carb (g)
1	TotFib (g)
3.35	Sugar (g)
0	SugAdd (g)
0.87	Fat (g)
0.11	SatFat (g)
0.23	MonoFat (g)
0.46	PolyFat (g)
0	TransFat (g)
0	Chol (mg)
25.49	Vit A-IU (IU)
5.19	Vit A-RAE (mcg)
1	Caroten (mcg)
4.69	Retinol (mcg)
5.92	BetaCaro (mcg)
0.04	Vit B1 (mg)
0.02	Vit B2 (mg)
0.19	Vit B3 (mg)
0.42	Vit B3-NE (mg)
0.02	Vit B6 (mg)
0.01	Vit B12 (mcg)
--	Biot (mcg)
20.62	Vit C (mg)
4.58	Vit D-IU (IU)
0.11	Vit D-mcg (mcg)

4.48	Vit E-a-Toco (mg)
4.98	Folate (mcg)
5.03	Vit K (mcg)
0.03	Panto (mg)
50.65	Calc (mg)
--	Chrom (mcg)
0.07	Copp (mg)
--	Fluor (mg)
--	Iodine (mcg)
0.42	Iron (mg)
12.33	Magn (mg)
0.24	Mang (mg)
--	Moly (mcg)
31.76	Phos (mg)
95.2	Pot (mg)
0.67	Sel (mcg)
11.28	Sod (mg)
0.23	Zinc (mg)
0.06	Omega3 (g)
0.4	Omega6 (g)
1.11	Chln (mg)

Please Note, nutritional vaules of all recipes may vary depending on the type of ingredients used "Nutritional analysis from Food Processor® Nutrition and Fitness Software version 11.5, ©2018 ESHA Research, Inc."

Endnotes:

[1] "Tips for Parents of Young Vegans" Reed Mangels PhD RD The Vegetarian Resource Group
[2] "Tips on Feeding Picky Toddlers" Dietitians of Canada
[3] Food Sources of B12 Dietitians of Canada
[4] Food Sources of Zinc Dietitians of Canada
[5] Food Sources of Iron Dietitians of Canada
[6] Nutrition Hotline Reed Mangels PhD RD The Vegetarian Resource Group
[7] Food Sources of Omega 3 Fats Dietitians of Canada
[8] Food Sources of Vitamin D Dietitians of Canada
[9] Food Source of Calcium Dietitians of Canada
[10] Food Sources of Iodine Dietitians of Canada
[11] "Vegan Weaning" Reed Mangels PhD RD, YouTube
[12] "Veganism in a Nutshell" The Vegetarian Resource Group
[13] "Do Canadian Children Meet Their Nutrient Requirements Through Food Intake Alone?" Health Canada
[14] "Dietary Reference Intake Tables" Health Canada
[15] Canadian Nutrient File Health Canada: Comparing Breast, Cow, and Goat's Milk Protein Content
[16] Food Sources of Folate Dietitians of Canada
[17] U.S. Department of Health and Human Services. National Institutes of Health

Sources Consulted:

"Tips for Parents of Young Vegan" Reed Mangels PhD RD The Vegetarian Resource Group
Date accessed March 26, 2018
http://www.vrg.org/family/tips_for_young_vegans.php

"Tips on Feeding Picky Toddlers" Dietitians of Canada
Date accessed March 26, 2018
https://www.dietitians.ca/Your-Health/Nutrition-A-Z/Toddlers/Tips-on-Feedy-Picky-Toddler.aspx

Food Sources of B12 Dietitians of Canada
Date accessed September 10, 2018
https://www.dietitians.ca/getattachment/45413d68-0639-4ad6-8de6-10eb97556e5f/FACTSHEET-Food-Sources-of-Vitamin-B12.pdf.aspx

Food Sources of Zinc Dietitians of Canada
Date accessed September 13, 2018
https://www.dietitians.ca/getattachment/e7b8fc00-09ad-4d4e-860a-eb9722f21adf/FACTSHEET-Food-Sources-of-Zinc.pdf.aspx

Food Sources of Iron Dietitians of Canada
Date accessed September 10, 2018
https://www.dietitians.ca/Downloads/Factsheets/Food-Sources-of-Iron.aspx

Nutrition Hotline Reed Mangels PhD RD The Vegetarian Resource Group
Date accessed September 20, 2018
https://www.vrg.org/journal/vj2016issue1/2016_issue1_nutrition_hotline.php

Food Sources of Omega 3 Fats Dietitians of Canada
Date accessed September 13, 2018

https://www.dietitians.ca/getattachment/de95e92c-3fb3-40db-b457-173de89bdc3a/FACTSHEET-Food-Sources-of-Omega-3-Fats.pdf.aspx

Food Sources of Vitamin D Dietitians of Canada
Date accessed September 10, 2018
https://www.dietitians.ca/getattachment/464f3006-0bb2-4f1a-a338-0b21d148bacb/FACTSHEET-Food-Sources-of-Vitamin-D.pdf.aspx

Food Sources of Calcium Dietitians of Canada
Date accessed September 13, 2018
https://www.dietitians.ca/getattachment/f739d485-d113-4a46-8122-eb2d33730c64/FACTSHEET-Food-Sources-of-Calcium.pdf.aspx

Food Sources of Iodine Dietitians of Canada
Date accessed September 13, 2018
https://www.dietitians.ca/Downloads/Factsheets/Food-Sources-of-Iodine.aspx

"Vegan Weaning" Reed Mangels, PhD RD YouTube
Date accessed March 26, 2018
https://www.youtube.com/watch?v=1yHJ2DsGHuo

"Veganism in a Nutshell" The Vegetarian Resource Group
Dated accessed March 26, 2018
http://www.vrg.org/nutshell/vegan.htm#nut

"Do Canadian Children Meet Their Nutrient Requirements Through Food Intake Alone?" Health Canada
Date accessed March 21, 2018
https://www.canada.ca/en/health-canada/services/food-nutrition/food-nutrition-surveillance/health-nu-trition-surveys/canadian-community-health-survey-cchs/canadian-children-meet-their-nutrient-require-ments-through-food-intake-alone-health-canada-2012.html

Dietary Reference Intake Tables Health Canada
Date accessed March 26, 2018
https://www.canada.ca/en/health-canada/services/food-nutrition/healthy-eating/dietary-reference-in-takes/tables.html

Canadian Nutrient File Health Canada: Comparing Breast, Cow, and Goat's Milk Protein Content
Date accessed September 13, 2018
https://food-nutrition.canada.ca/cnf-fce/report-rapport.do
https://food-nutrition.canada.ca/cnf-fce/report-rapport.do
https://food-nutrition.canada.ca/cnf-fce/report-rapport.do

Food Sources of Folate Dietitians of Canada
Date accessed September 13, 2018
https://www.dietitians.ca/getattachment/8612a7a9-642d-42dd-8e38-33f908c26c6a/FACTSHEET-Food-Sources-of-Folate.pdf.aspx

U.S. Department of Health and Human Services National Institutes of Health
Date accessed September 20, 2018
https://ods.od.nih.gov/factsheets/Iodine-HealthProfessional/#h3

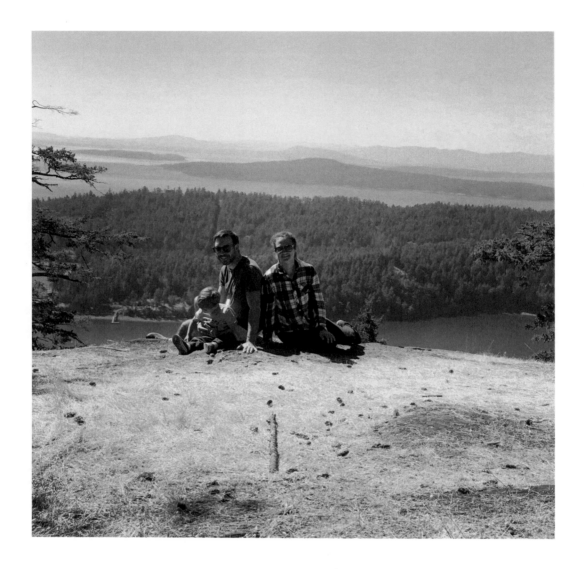

AMY HAMILTON is a health and wellness advocate, food photographer, and creator of www.canieatatrivers.com. She and her partner, Chad Mitchell, want to support and help families navigate their way around planning and preparing healthy and fun plant-based meals.

CHAD MITCHELL is an award-winning international Executive Chef. He now works full-time designing recipes and catering for Can I Eat At River's?.

RIVER MITCHELL is the ultimate recipe tester and not afraid to share his likes and dislikes.

Amy, Chad, and River live in the orchard and vineyard-filled Okanagan Valley in British Columbia, Canada. Go to www.canieatatrivers.com for products and services.